GENETICS OF EPILEPSY:
A REVIEW

Genetics of Epilepsy:
A Review

Michael E. Newmark, M.D.
and
J. Kiffin Penry, M.D.

Epilepsy Branch
Neurological Disorders Program
National Institute of Neurological and Communicative
Disorders and Stroke
National Institutes of Health
Bethesda, Maryland

Raven Press ■ New York

Raven Press, 1140 Avenue of the Americas, New York, New York 10036

Made in the United States of America

Library of Congress Cataloging in Publication Data

Newmark, Michael E
    Genetics of epilepsy.

    Includes bibliographic references and index.
    1. Epilepsy — Genetic aspects. I. Penry, J. Kiffin,
1929–   joint author. II. Title. [DNLM: 1. Epilepsy
—Familial and genetic. WL385 N556g]
RC372.N46   616.8'53'042   79–53067
ISBN 0–89004–394–9

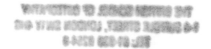

Preface

The hereditability of epilepsy is a crucial question for the epileptic patient who wishes to have children or for the parent of an epileptic child who wishes to have other children, and it can be a difficult question for the physician to answer. The risk varies widely according to the seizure type, the cause of the seizure disorder, and the sex and age of the epileptic patient. The genetics of epilepsy may suggest to the investigator an undisclosed underlying metabolic cause of a seizure disorder, and the identification of genetic forms of epilepsy may be a first clue to a metabolic etiology of the seizures.

In spite of the importance of the genetics of epilepsy, a consistent and coherent approach to the subject has not been formulated. Many of the current data are contradictory, and several significant clinical problems remain to be solved, including methods for the identification of relatives at highest risk for epilepsy, the effect of a family history of epilepsy on the prognosis of the seizure disorder, and the significance of the complex interactions of epilepsy, heredity, age, and hormonal and environmental factors. For example, why do absence seizures begin in childhood and largely subside after puberty? Are these genetically controlled age-specific manifestations? Or, does the developing nervous system determine the manifestations of seizures? These and many other questions need to be posed more clearly in view of new knowledge of the developing nervous system and new techniques for measuring hormonal and enzyme activities in the central nervous system.

This monograph attempts to provide a comprehensive review of the genetics of epilepsy, outlining what is currently known and suggesting where further information is required. It provides an extensive source of background information on the subject for investigators and for clinicians who treat epileptic patients, and should stimulate further evaluation of some of the unanswered questions about the inheritance of epilepsy.

Michael E. Newmark
J. Kiffin Penry
October 1979

Acknowledgments

We gratefully acknowledge the constructive criticisms of Dr. V. Elving Anderson and Dr. W. Allen Hauser. We also appreciate the assistance of the many members of the Epilepsy Branch who helped provide the source material and technical assistance that this review required.

Contents

I.

Introduction

Speculations on the hereditability of epilepsy have occupied the thoughts of medical men since the time of the earliest medical investigations. In approximately 450 B.C. the Greek physician Hippocrates concluded in his treatise *The Sacred Disease* that epilepsy is neither sacred nor even unexplainable; instead, it is inherited (as, indeed, are all diseases). The seat of the disease, he stated, is in the brain, which overflows with phlegm that clogs the veins and causes convulsions. Medieval Arabian physicians shared Hippocrates' conviction that the disorder had a hereditary basis. By the 16th century, epilepsy was so commonly accepted as an inherited malfunction that the English playwright John Haywood could mention heredity as a cause of epilepsy in *The Playe Called the Foure PP.*

One consequence of viewing epilepsy as an inherited disease was a Swedish law passed in 1757 that forbade epileptics to marry (Lundin and Miller, 1951), notwithstanding that epilepsy was known to combine with genius in such men as Julius Caesar. As a further and perhaps final step along this line of reasoning, the Nazi regime sterilized epileptics. Although the laws permitting these practices have been repealed, the question of the genetics of epilepsy remains open. An answer is needed for epileptics who wish to have children, as well as for susceptible family members.

However, in spite of the long history of a hereditary etiology of epilepsy, reliable scientific data either confirming or refuting the allegation have not been easy to obtain. Five factors make it difficult to establish the genetics of epilepsy:

1

1. In early clinical investigations, medical practitioners often did not agree on how to define epilepsy. Thus, hysteria and other paroxysmal disorders, including syncopy and vascular headache, were grouped with the epileptiform diseases. In addition, investigators were undecided as to whether single seizures and febrile convulsions should be included. Therefore, the baseline epilepsy rate in a community as well as the epilepsy rate of relatives could vary according to the definition of epilepsy used (Skre, 1978).

2. Seizures may occasionally be misdiagnosed, particularly when they are absence attacks or complex partial seizures which may be ignored or not considered to be epilepsy.

3. An inaccurate family history may be given, for several reasons. Sometimes sufficient medical information simply is not available concerning relatives beyond the immediate family, or families may attempt to conceal the potentially embarrassing disease by not reporting it. Even when information is supplied, a different number of relatives may be documented or the degree of relationship between the epileptic and other members of the family may not be included in the medical history.

4. An accurate diagnosis of epilepsy is often difficult because several unrelated conditions such as infections and metabolic disorders may be accompanied by seizures. Also, as will be discussed later, epilepsy can be a symptom of several hereditary diseases, both metabolic and degenerative. If patients with these diseases are included in a small series of accurately diagnosed epileptic patients, the hereditability of epilepsy may be exaggerated.

5. Finally, as noted by Lennox (1933), multiple contributing factors must be taken into account in the development of a seizure disorder. Although a genetic tendency toward epilepsy may exist, seizures may not occur unless factors such as stress, hormonal change, or numerous other environmental or physical triggers are present. Thus, patients who do not exhibit identifiable electroencephalographic abnormalities and who are not known to have seizures may nevertheless carry an epilepsy trait (Metrakos and Metrakos, 1961b). On the other hand, patients may be diagnosed as epileptics on the basis of electroencephalographic abnormalities that are later found to be the result of age, sex, alertness, or various environmental factors instead.

II.

Inheritance of Epilepsy: Indirect Evidence

Several recent studies have provided evidence that epilepsy is inherited. Although some of these data are not entirely convincing, they do at least suggest that epilepsy has a hereditary etiology.

A. NONSPECIFIC FAMILIAL ELECTRO-ENCEPHALOGRAPHIC PATTERNS

Nonspecific electroencephalographic patterns apparently can have genetic significance. One of them, the photoconvulsive response, has been extensively investigated and has been reviewed separately (Newmark and Penry, 1979). The spike-and-wave complex and the temporal-central spike, which are also patterns associated with epilepsy, will be discussed later. Electroencephalographic patterns that have not been as closely connected with epilepsy as the ones above are important nevertheless, because they suggest that cerebral electrical organization, at least as measured by the electroencephalogram, may be partially inherited.

That electroencephalographic patterns are influenced by nonspecific hereditary traits was noted by Lennox et al. (1945) during an early investigation of nonepileptic twins. Electroencephalograms from 85% of 55 monozygotic twin pairs were considered to be identical, in contrast to only 5% of the electroencephalograms from 19 dizygotic twin pairs. Although the determination of zygosity that was used in this study was not as specific as the blood-group assays available today, the investigators managed to separate the tracings accurately. Evoked-potential studies in twins have also supplied evidence supporting a generalized hereditary tendency of cerebral electrical organization. When the averaged visual-evoked potential (Dustman and Beck, 1965) and auditory-evoked potential (Rust, 1975) were applied, a higher correlation was found between monozygotic twin pairs than between the dizygotic ones. Lykken et al. (1974) examined monozygotic as well as dizygotic twin pairs using electroencephalographic frequency spectra and discovered that 96% of the monozygotic twins' electroencephalograms identically matched their co-twins'.

Another nonspecific familial electroencephalographic pattern is the 14- and 6/sec positive spikes, which is a pattern of uncertain clinical significance (Table 1). The 14- and 6/sec positive spikes are frequently present in relatives of epileptics and occur in siblings at a rate of about 50% (Rodin, 1964; Petersen and Akesson, 1968). Although the rate in siblings was lower in the Rodin sample, two-thirds of the patients had a close family member (parents, siblings, or offspring) diagnosed as having the pattern. The rate of parents affected was significantly

TABLE 1. *Familial nonspecific EEG patterns*

Pattern	Investigator	Mode of inheritance
Abnormal theta rhythm in childhood	Doose et al., 1967 Doose et al., 1972a	Multifactorial
Photoconvulsive reaction	Doose and Gerken, 1973	Multifactorial
Occipital 2–4/sec rhythm	Gerken and Doose, 1972	?
4–5 cycles/sec rhythm	Kuhlo et al., 1969	?
14– and 6/sec positive spike	Rodin, 1964 Petersen and Akes-son, 1968	? Autosomal dominant?
Frontal precentral beta	Vogel, 1966a	Autosomal dominant
Diffuse beta	Vogel, 1966a	?
Alpha variant of Vogel	Vogel, 1966b	Autosomal dominant

lower than that of siblings, suggesting that the 14- and 6/sec positive spike pattern, which is similar to the photoconvulsive response and the spike-and-wave discharge pattern, is age dependent.

Doose et al. (1972) described another hereditary pattern that is characterized by an abnormal theta rhythm consisting of monomorphic 4- to 6/sec waves that occur predominantly in the parietal regions. Abnormal theta rhythms appear most frequently in 3- and 4-year-old children. Of the patients manifesting this pattern, almost 29% of their siblings in the 3-to-4-year-old age group were also found to have theta rhythms, a rate approximately twice that of control children. The relation of this pattern to seizure activity is unclear, but the etiology of theta rhythms appears to be multifactorial.

Kuhlo et al. (1969) described a 4- to 5/sec rhythm that is seen in older individuals and present in the occipital-temporal areas; it was found in 10% of the siblings of affected probands. Clinically, the probands suffered from a wide variety of neurological symptoms, and several were nonepileptic. Gerken and Doose (1972) also noted occipital delta rhythms, most frequently in children under 10 years of age. Delta rhythms were present in 10% of the siblings of probands, which is a rate higher than that of the siblings of delta-negative patients but not higher than that of controls. The trait has little definite correlation with seizures.

Vogel and his colleagues published findings from several investigations that they conducted on a variety of familial patterns (Vogel, 1963; Vogel, 1966a; Vogel, 1966b; Vogel and Fujiya, 1969): generalized low-voltage activity, prominent alpha waves, continuous slow theta waves, frontal beta waves with high frequency and low voltage, almost continuous high voltage frontal-precentral theta waves, and diffuse beta waves. The researchers usually traced these patterns in several pedigrees, and they concluded from the results that the patterns were inherited. However, the hereditary aspects of the patterns remain controversial because such possible variables as medication, alertness, and accuracy of the records may have been responsible for them. A correlation with epilepsy has not been found, as is the case for many of the other patterns. The mode of inheritance appears to be autosomal dominant.

CHAPTER TWO

B. INHERITANCE OF EPILEPSY IN ANIMALS

Rodents with Audiogenic Seizures

The convulsive susceptibility of several rodents, including rabbits, mice, and rats, to auditory stimuli has been well described (Hall, 1947; Hirayama, 1963; Schlesinger et al., 1965; Horak, 1966; Wada and Ikeda, 1966; Wada, 1967; Hohenboken and Nellhaus, 1970; Boggan and Seiden, 1971; Kolpakov and Galaktionov, 1973; Hertz et al., 1974).

Different genetic models of seizure inheritance in audiogenic seizure-sensitive rats and rabbits have been postulated, such as a single gene with a pair of alleles, a threshold character that conceals underlying genetic variation, or multiple genes (Horak, 1966; Hohenboken and Nellhaus, 1970). As is the case for man, multiple environmental and physical factors affect the expression of the genes, including breeding cycles (Hall, 1947; Horak, 1966), the interval between litters (Horak, 1966), the incidence of seizures in the mother (Horak, 1966), and the age of the affected animal (Hertz et al., 1974).

In an effort to find a specific biochemical change that would explain the rodents' susceptibility to seizures, sodium-potassium-activated ATPase, norepinephrine, and serotonin levels were measured in the rodents, and methionine sulfoxamine, L-DOPA, reserpine, iproniazid, eserine, atropine, and thiosemicarbazide were administered to them to determine if an increase in neurotransmitters, neurotransmitter agonists, or neurotransmitter antagonists caused seizures. An exact explanation of the animals' susceptibility to seizures did not emerge from such experiments.

However, changes in the levels of some neurotransmitters have been shown to affect seizures. For example, brain serotonin and norepinephrine levels are lowest in the most seizure-prone animals at their most vulnerable age (Schlesinger et al., 1965), and the increased seizure susceptibility provoked by reserpine is reversed by L-3,4-dihydroxyphenyl-alanine (DOPA). When brain levels of dopamine are elevated, the seizure susceptibility is minimal (Boggan and Seiden, 1971). Wada and Ikeda (1966) noted the presence of audiogenic seizures in previously seizure-free rats who had been treated with methionine sulfoxamine, an analog of methionine. DOPA added to methionine sulfoxamine slightly potentiates its effect (Wada, 1969), but 5-HTP strongly inhibits the running phase of the seizure. Iproniazid, which strongly inhibits the running and the opisthotonic convulsions, is less effective if given half an hour after methionine sulfoxamine. Because eserine potentiates the effect of methionine sulfoxamine, whereas atropine substantially inhibits it, a cholinergic mechanism may be involved. Thiosemicarbamazide (an inhibitor of GABA production that acts by depression of glutamic acid decarboxylase activity) also increases the running behavior, again suggesting that more than a cholinergic mechanism is responsible for inherited susceptibility to seizures in animals. However, the enzyme and neurochemical changes responsible for the seizure sensitivity are not known.

Kolpakov and Galaktionov (1973) observed that cerebral oxidative phosphorylation appears to be altered in audiogenic seizure-sensitive rats and mice and have suggested that the polygenic inheritance of both species produced the biochemical alterations responsible for the sensitivity. Since the mechanisms of inheritance have not been fully documented in the audiogenic-seizure animals, the theory of polygenic inheritance may or may not explain the sensitivity to seizures exhibited by them.

Other Seizure-Susceptible Species

Hegreberg and Padgett (1976) described a familial progressive form of epilepsy in beagles that closely resembles progressive myoclonic epilepsy (Lafora's disease) with intracytoplasmic inclusions. In addition to this type, certain beagle colonies studied by Bielefeldt et al. (1971) have an increased tendency toward spontaneous convulsive seizures that is higher in males; a specific genetic mechanism, however, has not been discovered. The seizure trait is similarly sex modified in the British Alsatian, with more males than females affected, and with more than one gene involved (Falco et al., 1974). A genetic study of Keeshonds that relied on the use of electroencephalograms demonstrated a nonspe-

TABLE 2. Animals with increased seizure tendency

Animal	Seizure stimulus	Mode of inheritance	Investigator
Brown-Swiss cattle	Spontaneous	Autosomal dominant	Akesson et al., 1944
Beagle	Spontaneous	Uncertain	Bielefelt et al., 1971
	Spontaneous, light-induced	Uncertain	Hegreberg and Padgett, 1976
Mouse	Audiogenic seizure	Simple inheritance—dominant vs. recessive?	Collins and Fuller, 1968
		Uncertain	Hall, 1947
		Polygenetic	Kolpakov and Galaktionov, 1973
Mongolian gerbil	Spontaneous	Uncertain	Cox and Lomax, 1976
Chicken	Photic-induced, spontaneous	Autosomal recessive	Crawford, 1970
Deer mouse	Waltzing and audiogenic	Autosomal recessive	Dice, 1935
British Alsatian	Spontaneous	Polygenetic	Falco et al., 1974
Mouse-*ep*	See-saw motion	Autosomal dominant	Hirayama, 1963
		Autosomal dominant	Kurokawa et al., 1966
Rabbit	Audiogenic	Uncertain	Hohenboken and Nellhaus, 1970

Rat	Audiogenic	Uncertain	Horak, 1966
	Audiogenic	Polygenetic	Kolpakov and Galaktionov, 1973
Baboon *(Papio papio)*	Spontaneous, light-induced	Uncertain	Naquet and Lanoir, 1973
Swine	Spontaneous	Uncertain	Saunders, 1952
	Spontaneous	Uncertain	Bielefelt et al., 1971
Irish setter	Spontaneous	Uncertain	Saunders, 1952
Guinea pig	Audiogenic	Recessive	Saunders, 1952
Keeshonds	Spontaneous	Uncertain	Wallace, 1975
Syrian golden hamster	Spontaneous	Autosomal recessive	Yoon et al., 1976

cific hereditary tendency that again is known to affect predominantly males (Wallace, 1975). The baboon *(Papio papio)* and the chicken suffer from photic-induced and spontaneous seizures (Newmark and Penry, 1979), and many animals suffer from other types of clinical attacks (Table 2). Other animals reviewed by Saunders (1952) exhibited a variety of seizure types and hereditary patterns.

Drugs that increase central dopamine activity without reducing norepinephrine activity reduce the severity of seizures in a seizure-sensitive strain of Mongolian gerbils (Cox and Lomax, 1976). Adenine nucleotide levels change and glutamic acid levels increase during different phases of induced convulsions in the *ep* mouse (Hirayama, 1963).

Summary

Several animal species are susceptible to seizures. In a few cases these observations have been correlated with neurochemical changes in the brain, particularly with changed levels of GABA and catecholamines; and with altered oxidative-phosphorylative metabolism. Specific biochemical abnormalities responsible for specific seizures, however, have not been demonstrated. Again, the evidence for the hereditability of epilepsy in humans is inconclusive, because several of the animal seizure types are only endemic in an individual species.

C. HEREDITARY DISEASES ASSOCIATED WITH EPILEPSY

Several hereditary diseases affecting the central nervous system have been associated with epilepsy. Although many of them occur quite rarely, a few are seen in appreciable numbers. In a small series of pedigrees, their significance may be exaggerated; however, they are important since they may suggest biochemical mechanisms by which the hereditary traits of epilepsy are expressed. Reviews of hereditary disorders associated with epilepsy have been conducted by Gastaut (1969), Green (1973), and Skre (1975).

Known Metabolic Disorders

Many metabolic disorders with known causes have been described in which seizures are either an early or an occasional symptom (Tables 3A–3E). Included in this category are disorders of amino acid metabolism and of lipid metabolism, glycogen storage diseases [Nos. 1 and 3, as well as UDPG-glycogen transferase deficiency (Menkes, 1974)], mucopolysaccharidosis, Hurler's and Hunter's diseases (Green, 1973), pyridoxine-dependency syndrome, Wilson's disease, and Menkes' kinky-hair syndrome. Generally these diseases are inherited as autosomal-recessive disorders, although a few are sex-linked (Hunter's disease and Menkes' kinky-hair syndrome), and one, hereditary coproporphyria, is dominant. They are usually associated with several other progressive neurological

TABLE 3A. *Hereditary diseases associated with epilepsy*

Disorders of amino acid metabolism	Mode of inheritance	Investigator
Histidinemia	Autosomal recessive	Duffner and Cohen, 1975
Carbamyl phosphate synthetase deficiency	Autosomal recessive	Hommes et al., 1969
Hyperprolinemia	Autosomal recessive	Menkes, 1974
Hyperlysinemia	?	Menkes, 1974
Hyper-beta-alaninemia	?	Menkes, 1974
Carnosinemia	?	Menkes, 1974
Lactic acidemia	?	Menkes, 1974
Arginosuccinic aciduria	Autosomal recessive	Radermecker and Dumon, 1969
Homocystinuria	Autosomal recessive	Radermecker and Dumon, 1969
Maple-syrup urine disease	Autosomal recessive	Radermecker and Dumon, 1969
Phenylketonuria	Autosomal recessive	Szabo et al., 1965

TABLE 3B. *Hereditary diseases associated with epilepsy*

Disorders of carbohydrate metabolism	Mode of inheritance	Investigator
Glycogen storage disease I (glucose 6-phosphatase deficiency)	Autosomal recessive	Menkes,1974
Glycogen storage disease III (amylo-1,6 glucosidase and/or oligo 1,4-1,4 glucan-transferase deficiency)	Autosomal recessive	Menkes, 1974
UDPG-glycogen transferase deficiency	Autosomal recessive	Menkes, 1974

TABLE 3C. *Hereditary diseases associated with epilepsy*

Disorders of lipid metabolism	Mode of inheritance	Investigator
G_{M1} gangliosidosis (familial neurovisceral lipidosis)	Autosomal recessive	Green, 1973
Globoid cell leukodystrophy (Krabbe's disease)	Autosomal recessive	Green, 1973
Metachromatic leukodystrophy (cerebroside sulfatidosis)	Autosomal recessive	Green, 1973
Glucocerebrosidosis (Gaucher's disease)	Autosomal recessive	Green, 1973
Sphingomyelinase deficiency	Autosomal recessive	Green, 1973
G_{M2} gangliosidosis (Tay-Sach's disease)	Autosomal recessive	Menkes et al., 1971
Batten, Bielschowsky diseases	Autosomal recessive	Menkes et al., 1971
Spielmeyer-Vogt disease	Autosomal recessive	Menkes et al., 1971

TABLE 3D. *Hereditary diseases associated with epilepsy*

Mucopolysaccharidosis	Mode of inheritance	Investigator
Hurler's disease	Autosomal recessive	Green, 1973
Hunter's disease	Sex-linked recessive	Green, 1973

TABLE 3E. *Hereditary diseases associated with epilepsy*

Other metabolic diseases	Mode of inheritance	Investigator
Hepatolenticular degeneration (Wilson's disease)	Autosomal recessive	Green, 1973
Hereditary coproporphyria	Autosomal dominant	Houston et al., 1977
Menke's kinky hair syndrome	Sex-linked recessive	Menkes, 1974
Hyperfolic acidemia	?	Radermecker and Dumon, 1969
Pyridoxine-dependency syndrome	?	Radermecker and Dumon, 1969

deficits. With the exception of the pyridoxine-dependency syndrome, seizures are rarely the only prominent symptom of these disorders. Seizures are commonly diagnosed in them when typical clinical presentations occur or when biochemical tests are performed on a poorly developing child.

Progressive Myoclonic Epilepsies

In addition to the diseases that have a known metabolic disorder, seizures are a symptom of other degenerative disorders in which the metabolic defect has not yet been discovered (Table 3F). One of the most prominent of these disorders is progressive myoclonic epilepsy, or the group of progressive myoclonic epilepsies. Several hereditary

TABLE 3F. *Other hereditary or heredodegenerative diseases*

Disease	Mode of inheritance	Investigator
Scapulohumeral muscular dystrophy	Autosomal dominant?	Aschner et al., 1964
Hereditary ataxias	Variable	Andermann et al., 1976; Skre, 1975; Gayral and Gayral, 1969
Unverricht myoclonic epilepsy	Autosomal recessive	Barolin and Pateisky, 1969; Janeway et al., 1967; Quattrini et al., 1975
Leukodystrophy (type?)	Autosomal recessive	Bignami et al., 1966
Benign familial neonatal convulsions	Autosomal dominant	Bjerre and Corelius, 1968
Borjeson-Forssman-Lehmann syndrome	Sex-linked recessive	Borjeson et al., 1962
Genetic spastic oligophrenia and essential myoclonus	?	Book, 1953
Dysnergia cerebellaris myoclonia (Ramsay-Hunt syndrome)	Autosomal recessive	Diebold et al., 1974
Progressive, late amaurotic idiocy	Autosomal dominant	Dumon and Radermecker, 1965
Sudanophilic leukodystrophy (Pelizaeus-Merzbacher disease)	Sex-linked recessive	Green, 1973
Adrenal leukodystrophy	Sex-linked recessive	Green, 1973
Alexander's disease	?	Green, 1973
Hereditary hematuria	Autosomal recessive	Hirooka et al., 1969
Norrie's disease	Autosomal recessive	Jancar, 1970

Disease	Inheritance	Reference
Lloyd's disease	?	Kramer and Makkink, 1961
Familial essential myoclonus	?	Korten et al., 1974
Canavan's sclerosis	Autosomal recessive	Mirimanoff, 1976
Infantile familial epileptogenous encephalopathy	Autosomal recessive?	Pescia, 1973
Brachmetapodia	Autosomal dominant?	Poch et al., 1976
Von Hippel–Lindau's disease	Autosomal dominant	Radermecker and Dumon, 1969
Tuberous sclerosis	Autosomal dominant	Radermecker and Dumon, 1969
Sturge-Weber disease	Autosomal dominant	Radermecker and Dumon, 1969
Neurofibromatosis	Autosomal dominant	Radermecker and Dumon, 1969
Huntington's chorea	Autosomal dominant	Schiottz-Christensen, 1969
Paine syndrome	Sex-linked recessive	Seemanova et al., 1973
Charcot-Marie-Tooth disease	Variable	Skre, 1975
Roussy-Levy disease	Variable	Skre, 1975
Marinesco-Sjogren syndrome	Variable	Skre, 1975
Hereditary spastic paraplegia	Variable	Skre, 1975; Malin, 1976
Miscellaneous myoclonic epilepsies	Mixed	Several authors
Hartung myoclonic epilepsy	Autosomal recessive	Vogel, 1969
Lundborg myoclonic epilepsy	Autosomal recessive	Vogel, 1969; Stern and Eldridge, 1973
Muscular dystrophy (Fukuyama type)	Autosomal recessive	Segawa, 1976
Oster-Weber-Rendu disease	Autosomal	Weiss and Badurowa, 1967

forms of this syndrome have been described; thus, since the underlying defect is not known, the syndrome may prove to be a group of disorders rather than a specific disease.

The myoclonic epilepsies have been organized into four types: (1) the Unverricht type, characterized by recessive inheritance, a severe course, early death, and a Lafora body; (2) the Lundborg type, character- ized by recessive inheritance and similar pathological findings but a much slower course; (3) the Hartung type, associated with autosomal- dominant inheritance and a variable course; and (4) an unclassifiable variable group (Vogel et al., 1965; Vogel, 1969). Occasionally both the fast (Unverricht) and the slow (Lundborg) forms may be found in the same family (Buscaino et al., 1973). Diebold (1972) maintained the first three categories in his classification of the myoclonic epilepsies but added a new type: progressive myoclonic epilepsy, identifiable by degenerative changes in the central nervous system, a slow progression, low-grade symptoms, and an autosomal-recessive inheritance. Essen- tially similar classifications were used by Stern and Eldridge (1973), modified by the additional discovery that the autosomal-dominant type is usually characterized by sensory neural hearing loss.

Other investigators, however, have noted individual families and pa- tients with myoclonic epilepsy syndromes that do not quite fit the above schemes of classification. Gross-Sellback and Doose (1975) and Shiba- saki et al. (1973) described families with myoclonus present primarily during wakefulness, which increased with anxiety but took a benign course during normal living. Occasionally myoclonic seizures are associ- ated with what is probably a metabolic disorder. Klein et al. (1968a, 1968b) reported myoclonic epilepsy and retinitis pigmentosa in a Valais family, in which one member was found to have PAS-positive inclusions in several organs at autopsy. The progressive myoclonic syndrome was observed in a woman exhibiting a retinal cherry red spot (Guazzi et al., 1973), whose liver biopsy and urinary studies suggested a polymuco- saccharidosis. Chiofalo et al. (1974) reported patients suffering from progressive myoclonic epilepsy who had elevated plasma iron determina- tions and iron present in the central nervous system as well as in various organs. Several of these familial syndromes in association with myoclonic seizures suggest well-delineated, or specific, diseases.

Hereditary Ataxias

The hereditary ataxias and related disorders, including Charcot-Marie-Tooth disease, Roussy-Levy disease, and hereditary spastic paraplegia, have also been associated with epilepsy. Gayral and Gayral (1969) noted that 9% of 67 members from 8 families that had a hereditary ataxia also had seizures, as did 22% of the 13 neurologically impaired individuals. Seizures associated with Friedrich's ataxia were analyzed by Andermann et al. (1976), who found that 6.9% of the 58 affected individuals had seizures, as did 4.3% of the parents and 2.7% of the siblings. The investigators concluded that epilepsy may be inherited either secondary to a multifactorial inheritance separate from Friedrich's ataxia or secondary to the abnormalities caused by the ataxia gene itself.

Other Disorders

A wide variety of neuroectodermal diseases that are frequently associated with epilepsy are usually secondary either to a cortical tumor or to angiomatosis. Among these are neurofibromatosis, tuberous sclerosis, Osler-Weber-Rendu disease, von Hippel-Lindau's disease, and Sturge-Weber's disease. Poch et al. (1970) described a family of 15 individuals spanning three generations who were afflicted with abnormalities of the hands and feet, some of whom also exhibited seizures.

Epilepsy associated with prominent endocrine abnormalities was noted by Borjeson et al. (1962), and families with epilepsy, various endocrine abnormalities, and mental deficiencies that were transmitted by an X-linked recessive gene were reported by Barr and Galindo (1965). Ioanitiu et al. (1966) observed a combination of epilepsy and thyropathic endemic dystrophy, which they interpreted to be secondary to a genetic epileptic tendency that was enhanced by a thyroid abnormality. A simi-

17

lar combination of factors was also described by Kramer and Makkink (1961) in a family with epilepsy and multiple endocrine adenomas. Although epilepsy, multiple tumors, and mental retardation were present in the patient's family, the single autopsy demonstrated primarily hippocampal changes consistent with hypoglycemia as the etiology of the index patient's epilepsy.

Schiottz-Christensen (1969) examined a pair of monozygotic twins who exhibited generalized tonic-clonic seizures and Huntington's disease; subsequently, he found other examples of epilepsy associated with Huntington's disease cited in the literature. When one takes into account that dopaminergic alterations are known to occur in this disease, that several antiepileptic agents have extrapyramidal side effects, and that agents producing extrapyramidal effects often change the seizure threshold of experimental models and epileptic patients, the possibility that an interrelation exists among dopamine levels, the occurrence of epilepsy, and genetic inheritance in Huntington's disease has some factual support.

The association of a hereditary familial tremor with epilepsy was discovered by Wakeno (1975), who reported 14 individuals of a 35-member family that had a history of hereditary tremor and clinical seizures extending through five generations. Aschner et al. (1964) provided a pedigree of persons having either scapulohumeral dystrophy or generalized tonic-clonic seizures. Other degenerative diseases, including Norrie's disease (a sex-linked recessive oculocerebral degeneration) and Paine's syndrome (a sex-linked recessive microcephaly with spastic tetraplegia and mental retardation), may also be associated with epilepsy.

Summary

Numerous hereditary diseases are associated with epilepsy. Several of these diseases do not have a known metabolic disorder, but the breadth of the resulting abnormalities that affect various anatomical and biochemical sites is so extensive that a direct correlation of epilepsy with a single metabolic factor is not yet possible. Most hereditary diseases associated with epilepsy have a widespread effect on the central nervous system, are linked with mental retardation and profound neurological defects, and often produce generalized seizures. Some hereditary disorders, including fibromatosis, tuberous sclerosis, and Sturge-Weber disease, produce seizures that are usually the result of a tumor or angioma; thus, they form a group separate from the generalized hereditary disorders. However, in actuality, the association of epilepsy with proven hereditary diseases may suggest a stronger probability of a genetic etiology for epilepsy than is warranted.

D. CHROMOSOMAL ABNORMALITIES ASSOCIATED WITH EPILEPSY

Only a few chromosomal abnormalities associated with epilepsy have been described (Table 4). Nielsen and Pedersen (1969) investigated patients who had either Klinefelter's or XYY syndrome and found that 15% of the 33 patients had a history of epilepsy, and 26% of the 31 patients tested had abnormal electroencephalograms. Patients with chromosome 47 XYY were found by Benezech et al. (1972) and Benezech and Noel (1975) to have epilepsy; however, Forssman and Akesson (1969) did not find a chromosomal XYY abnormality in the epileptic patients they studied.

Dobson and Ohnuki (1961) noted secondary constrictions in chromosomes of a 6-year-old child with epilepsy, Kunze et al. (1975) found

TABLE 4. *Chromosomal abnormalities possibly associated with seizure disorders*

Disorder	Investigator
XYY	Benezech and Noel, 1975
XXY (Klinefelter's syndrome)	Nielsen and Pedersen, 1969
XXX (Triple X women)	Radermecker and Dumon, 1969
13–15 Trisomy	Radermecker and Dumon, 1969
21 Trisomy (Down's syndrome)	Radermecker and Dumon, 1969

a ring-shaped chromosome of the G group in a 10-year-old retarded girl who exhibited myoclonic seizures, and Frezza et al. (1966) described a family in which all of the members had an extra metacentric chromosome, with one member manifesting seizures as well. In view of the small number of these patients, however, an accurate correlation is not possible. Thus, no evidence definitely supports an association of epilepsy with chromosomal abnormalities.

III.

Inheritance of Epilepsy: Direct Evidence

A. CLINICAL STUDIES OF PROBANDS AND RELATIVES

The genetics of epilepsy have been studied most frequently with large-scale clinical investigations of the relatives of epileptics. Methods used to examine the relatives, type of relationship, criteria for a seizure disorder, reliability of data, and type of seizure documented have varied, which has resulted in a considerable spectrum of opinion on the question of whether heredity is an important factor in epilepsy or not. This ambiguity could continue to plague genetic investigations of epilepsy indefinitely, or at least until the metabolic etiologies of some of the epilepsies are precisely defined (Brady, 1976).

Reviews of the large-scale studies on the families of epileptics that include discussions of the conflicting data and some of the problems encountered in genetic investigations have been published by Kallman and Saunder (1947), Harvald (1951), Harvald (1954), Harvald (1958), Hurst (1963), Koch (1963), Delaveleye (1965), Inouye (1968), Ortiz de Zarote (1968), Gastaut (1969), Metrakos and Metrakos (1970), Beaussart (1971), Alvarez (1972), Metrakos and Metrakos (1972), Refsum (1972), Vercelletto (1972), and Hurst (1974).

Studies of Probands with Multiple-Seizure Types

The most commonly done study on the genetics of epilepsy has been examinations of the relatives of probands diagnosed as being multiple-seizure types. In this kind of study the results vary with the method used and the types of seizure included. For example, the data of Alstrom

(1950) indicated no significant hereditary cause of epilepsy, whereas Metrakos and Metrakos (1960) found a very significant hereditary effect (Table 5).

Studies Claiming No Hereditary Risk

The leading proponents of a nonhereditary or weakly hereditary cause of epilepsy have been Marburg and Helfand (1946), Sorel (1969), Beaussart and Loiseau (1969), Eisner et al. (1959), and Alstrom (1950). The Marburg and Helfand study, which reported that only 2% of 100 probands had a significant family history of seizures, involved probands with a mixture of several types and severity, and the relatives themselves were not examined. The Beaussart and Loiseau report (1969), which cited only 2.5% of 5,200 families as having more than one epileptic, is similarly flawed by a lack of specificity in the epileptics chosen for study and an absence of direct examination of the relatives, although in most of the families other means were found to corroborate the history. In the Sorel report (1969), only 1% of 2,488 patients with mixed seizures had a familial history of epilepsy, but the report did not mention how the relatives were studied. When the probands were restricted to 202 patients whose neurological examinations had proved normal but who had manifested generalized electroencephalographic abnormalities, 27% had a familial seizure history. Sorel's study thus seems to suggest a genetic cause of epilepsy in some patients rather than denying such an etiology.

Alstrom (1950) and Eisner et al. (1959) have conducted two of the more carefully done investigations on the genetics of epilepsy. Eisner and colleagues excluded febrile seizures and metabolically caused convulsions and investigated other seizure types. Although Eisner et al. (1959) state that a hereditary etiology cannot definitely be established from their large study of 669 epileptic patients and 3,362 close relatives, several familial trends were apparent. The most significant finding was that 8.3% of the close relatives of probands who had generalized tonic-seizures and whose seizures had begun before the age of 4 also had generalized tonic-clonic seizures, compared with 2.2% of the relatives

TABLE 5. *Multiple seizures—clinical evaluation*

| | Probands | | | | | Relatives | | | | | |
Investigator	Seizure type	No.	Sex	Age range	Percent with positive family history	Relationship	No.	Sex	Age range	Seizure type	Percent affected
Alstrom, 1950	Mixed, unknown etiology	606	M 306 F 300			Parents Siblings Offspring	1,207 2,237 548			All seizures including single seizures	1.7 1.9 4.0
						Parents Siblings Offspring	1,207 2,237 548			All seizures excluding single seizures	1.5 1.6 3.1
	Mixed, probable etiology known	150	M 92 F 58			Parents Siblings Offspring	285 470 135			All seizures including single seizures	1.8 1.2 5.4
						Parents Siblings Offspring	285 470 135			All seizures excluding single seizures	1.1 1.2 3.6
	Mixed, known etiology	141	M 94 F 47			Parents Siblings Offspring	272 555 142			All seizures including single seizures	1.2 1.5 3.2
						Parents Siblings Offspring	272 551 142			All seizures excluding single seizures	0.8 1.3 1.6
	Total	897	M 492 F 405			Parents Siblings Offspring	1,764 3,258 825			All seizures including single seizures	1.7 1.7 4.1

TABLE 5. (Continued)

Investigator	Probands — Seizure type	No.	Sex	Age range	Percent with positive family history	Relatives — Relationship	No.	Sex	Age range	Seizure type	Percent affected
Andermann, 1972	Patients with centrencephalic EEG pattern	336				Parents	1,764			All seizures excluding single seizures	1.4
						Siblings	3,258				1.5
						Offspring	825				2.7
						Close	999				17.9
						Parents	400				16.8
						Siblings	519				20.0
						Offspring	80				10.0
Annegers et al.,	Mixed	183	F			Offspring	351			Epilepsy, Febrile convulsions	2.8
											2.6
		108	M			Offspring	229			Epilepsy, Febrile convulsions	0.0
											1.3
			F	0–9 (onset)		Offspring	79			Epilepsy	3.8
			F	10–19		Offspring	124			Epilepsy	4.0
			F	>20		Offspring	152			Epilepsy	1.3
			F			Offspring	190	M		Epilepsy	3.2
										Febrile convulsions	3.2

Reference	Type	Probands, N (M / F)	Probands group / age	Probands %	Relationship	Relatives, N	Relatives sex	Relatives age	Outcome	%
Beaussart and Loiseau, 1969	Mixed, "generalized"	5,200 / 3,380	M	2.5 / 3.2	Offspring	165	F		Epilepsy / Febrile convulsions	2.4 / 2.4
Bridge, 1949	Mixed	742	Children	42.7	Offspring	138	M		Epilepsy / Febrile convulsions	0.0 / 2.2
Cobb, 1932	Secondary to head trauma	1,086 / 235			Offspring	96	F		Epilepsy / Febrile convulsions	0.0 / 0.0
					All	9,139				2.1 / 1.4
Conrad, 1937	Idiopathic epilepsy	155 / 151	M / F — 35–90		Offspring	994 (498 M, 496 F)	M / F	0–65	Epilepsy	6.0
	Intermediate epilepsy	96 / 38	M / F — 35–90		Offspring	442 (224 M, 218 F)	M / F	0–59	Epilepsy	2.7
Echeverria, 1880	Mixed	136 (62 M, 74 F)			Offspring	553			Infantile convulsions or epilepsy	49.0
						264 / 289	M / F			50.0 / 49.0

TABLE 5. *(Continued)*

	Probands					Relatives					
Investigator	Seizure type	No.	Sex	Age range	Percent with positive family history	Relation-ship	No.	Sex	Age range	Seizure type	Percent affected
Eisner et al., 1959	"Idiopathic"	321				Close	1,658			Convulsions all types	6.53
										Generalized tonic-clonic	5.26
										Other	1.27
	Mixed seizures (more than 1 type in 1 individual)	100				Close	457			Convulsions of all types	5.24
										Generalized tonic-clonic	4.65
Gaches et al., 1967	Mixed	1,100		14–18	7.8						
		1,150		>14	9.1						
Gowers, 1881	Mixed	1,218			35.0						
		584	M		33.0						
		634	F		37.0						
Harvald, 1951	Cryptogenic					Siblings	2,254	M		Epilepsy	3.73
						Siblings	2,314	F		Epilepsy	4.36
	Intermediate					Siblings	341	M		Epilepsy	1.56
						Siblings	330	F		Epilepsy	1.58
	Cryptogenic					Siblings	950	M		Epilepsy	2.76
						Siblings	962	F		Epilepsy	2.96

Author, year	Category	No. probands	Relatives	No. relatives	Disorder	%
	Intermediate	203	Siblings	84	Epilepsy	0.0
		237	Siblings	84	Epilepsy	2.28
		M 120		M		
		F 117		F		
Harvald, 1954	"Cryptogenic" All types		Near	829		3.5
			Distant	1,637		2.3
			Relatives of male probands	1,425		3.1
			Relatives of female probands	1,361		1.8
	Mixed, with markedly abnormal EEG	130	Near	503		4.3
			Distant	1,095		2.6
	Mixed, with normal or slightly abnormal EEG	41	Near	220		2.6
			Distant	310		2.0
	Focally abnormal EEG	66	Near	229		3.7
			Distant	429		1.2
	All types		Parents	469	Epilepsy	4.1
			Siblings	425	Epilepsy	3.4
			Offspring	58	Epilepsy	1.7
Kimball, 1954	Mixed, with 1 parent with epilepsy	294	Siblings	776	Epilepsy	13.5
	Mixed, without epileptic parent	222	Siblings	550	Epilepsy	9.5
Kruse, 1964	Seizures during sleep	115	Children	17.0		

TABLE 5. *(Continued)*

Investigator	Seizure type	Probands No.	Sex	Age range	Percent with positive family history	Relation-ship	Relatives No.	Sex	Age range	Seizure type	Percent affected
Lennox, 1947a	Mixed	2,130			17.0	Near	12,119				2.7
	Mixed, with normal exam					Near	10,152				3.0
	Mixed			0–4		Near	3,747				4.5
				5–19		Near	5,170				2.5
				>20		Near	4,497				1.2
Lennox, 1951	Mixed, with normal neuro-logical exam			0–1		Near	15,690			Epilepsy	3.6
				2–4		Near	2,125			Epilepsy	6.4
				5–9		Near	1,674			Epilepsy	5.7
				10–19		Near	2,319			Epilepsy	4.1
				20–29		Near	4,785			Epilepsy	3.1
						Near	2,543			Epilepsy	2.1
Lennox and Davis, 1950	Mixed, with 3 cps spike-and-wave	193			34.2						
	Mixed, with slow spike-and wave	187			27.2						

Study	Disorder	No. probands	Sex		Relative	No. relatives	Type	%
Metrakos and Metrakos, 1960	Convulsions	68			Parents	136	Convulsions	9.6
					Siblings	104	Convulsions	9.6
					Aunts and uncles	706	Convulsions	5.8
					Grandparents	272	Convulsions	1.5
					Cousins	1,022	Convulsions	1.7
					Total	2,240	Convulsions	3.8
Metrakos and Metrakos, 1961a	Seizure disorders	42	F		Parents	162	Convulsions	11.7
		39	M		Siblings	200	Convulsions	13.5
	Centrencephalic EEG (typical)				Aunts and uncles	790	Convulsions	4.2
					Grandparents	324	Convulsions	2.8
					Cousins	1,229	Convulsions	2.0
					Total	4,672		4.1
	Seizure disorder and atypical centrencephalic EEG	66	F		Parents	260	Convulsions	14.6
		64	M		Siblings	319	Convulsions	12.2
					Aunts and uncles	1,377	Convulsions	4.2
	Seizure disorder with centrencephalic EEG	108	F		Grandparents	520	Convulsions	2.5
		103	M		Cousins	2,196	Convulsions	1.2
					Total	4,672	Convulsions	3.72
					Mixed	4,065	Convulsions	3.84
					Mixed	3,312	Convulsions	3.93
Muskins, 1928	Mixed	2,000						
		1,000	M	31.1	All relatives			
		1,000	F	33.6	All relatives			

TABLE 5. *(Continued)*

	Probands						Relatives				
Investigator	Seizure type	No.	Sex	Age range	Percent with positive family history	Relationship	No.	Sex	Age range	Seizure type	Percent affected
Ounstead, 1952	Mixed, afebrile fits	106		Children	45.0						
	Mixed, including febrile fits	333		Children 0–1 1–2 3–5 >5	39.0 40.0 60.0 40.0 24.0	Siblings	490			"Convulsive disorder"	11.4
Paskind and Brown, 1936	Mixed, with normal or almost normal exam	266			7.5						
Paskind and Brown, 1936	Mixed, with normal or almost normal exam	162				Offspring	342		0–>25	Epilepsy Other seizure disorders	0.29 1.7
Paskind and Brown, 1937	Mixed, with normal and almost normal neurological exam	331			8.4						

Study	Type	N	Age	%	Relationship	N	Condition	%
Sallou and Poissonnier, 1969	Mixed	1,018	14–18	8.4	Parents		Infantile convulsions	14.2
Sasagawa, 1976	Mixed (in childhood)	125	Children	47.2				
Sorel, 1969	Mixed, idiopathic with normal exam	202		27.0			Seizure disorder	
	Symptomatic or pathological neurological exam			1.0			Seizure disorder	
Soulayrol et al., 1969	Mixed	1,600	0–18	14.25			Any convulsion	
		400	0–7	8.8			Epilepsy	
		900	7–14	9.3			Epilepsy	
		300	14–18	9.7			Epilepsy	
Stein, 1933	Mixed	1,000	1–75 (avg. 16–20)	27.4	Parents, siblings, and offspring	6,512	Seizure disorder	3.7
					Siblings	4,305		4.1
					Mothers	1,000		3.5
					Fathers	1,000		2.3
					Offspring	267		2.2

TABLE 5. *(Continued)*

	Probands					Relatives					
Investigator	Seizure type	No.	Sex	Age range	Percent with positive family history	Relation-ship	No.	Sex	Age range	Seizure type	Percent affected
Tanaka and Aramitsu, 1962	Mixed (without previous neurological disorder)	331 192 139	 M F		12.2						
Thom, 1915	"Hereditary epilepsy"	82 75	F M		57.0						
Thom, 1916	Mixed	33 13 20	 M F			Offspring	133			Seizure disorder	7.5
Thom, 1922	Mixed	117 76 41	 F M			Offspring	431			Seizure disorder	7.7
Tsuboi and Endo, 1977	Mixed	121	M			Offspring	233			Seizure disorder	6.9
		142	F			Offspring	273			Seizure disorder	11.0
		263				Offspring	506			Seizure disorder	9.1

Study	Seizure type	N	Age	Relationship	N	Sex	Age	Outcome	%
				Offspring	233	M		Seizure disorder	6.9
				Offspring	273	F		Seizure disorder	11.0
				Offspring	149	M + F	0–4	Seizure disorder	5.4
				Offspring	96	M + F	5–9	Seizure disorder	10.4
				Offspring	68	M + F	10–14	Seizure disorder	11.8
				Offspring	49	M + F	15–19	Seizure disorder	16.3
				Offspring	144	M + F	>20	Seizure disorder	8.3
	Mixed	35	0–4	Offspring	63			Seizure disorder	20.6
		82	5–19	Offspring	143			Seizure disorder	4.2
		146	>20	Offspring	300			Seizure disorder	9.0
Van den Berg, 1974	Mixed	65	Childhood	Siblings (older)	152			Convulsions	6.6
				Siblings (younger)	47			Convulsions	6.3

of control patients. This contrast to controls is even more significant because the control patients were selected from diabetes, rheumatism, and hearing and speech clinics, and therefore had familial diseases that are often associated with epilepsy or other neurological disorders. Although relatives of unselected epileptic patients did not have a significantly increased seizure history (5.24% compared with 2.69% of controls), the prevalence of epilepsy in these controls was higher than in other studies, possibly reflecting the selection of the controls. The failure to include infantile or febrile seizures in the epileptic group may also have reduced the prominence of the contrast.

Alstrom extensively studied the relatives of 897 unselected epilepsy patients from the only neurology university clinic in Sweden at that time. The parents, siblings, and offspring of this mixed group of patients were examined for a history of epilepsy. The examination usually consisted of interviews with the relatives who lived at the home of the proband. The relatives who were not living with the proband were investigated by means of any available records. Although only 1.7% of the relatives of patients having epilepsy of unknown etiology had seizures, and only 1.1% of the relatives of patients with a known etiology had seizures, the seizure rate of the relatives in this study is much higher if the youngest age group is analyzed, and if relatives who had experienced single seizures are considered. When single epileptic attacks are included, 4.1% of the offspring of epileptic patients had seizures. Since the probands included all types of seizure patients, and since the age of the relatives was not specifically analyzed (except in terms of a relationship; for example, offspring, sibling, or parent, which gives a rough estimate of age), this investigation may not conflict with studies that indicate a definite hereditary correlation. Thus, even the studies claiming no hereditary risk suggest an increased risk in close relatives, particularly in patients who have a seizure disorder of unknown etiology or of a generalized type.

Studies Supporting a Hereditary Risk

Some of the studies that presume epilepsy is definitely correlated with genetic inheritance are also unspecific. Many of the early investigators broadly defined epilepsy and counted nonseizure events such as attacks of an "insane nature" as epilepsy (Echeverria, 1880). Although these attacks may have been complex partial seizures at that, no further description was given. Gowers (1881) grouped hysterical seizures as a type of epilepsy, and Muskens (1928) included migraine in his epilepsy histories. Criteria for categorizing disorders as epilepsy, specific details concerning the methods of investigation of relatives, and even the number of relatives examined were often not stated in these early works.

Offspring data. Several investigators have found that the offspring of epileptic patients have a higher than expected seizure rate. Thom and Walker (1922) found that 7.7% of 431 offspring from epileptic parents had either suffered convulsions in infancy or had developed epilepsy at some later time. Fifteen percent of the fathers and 21% of the 76 mothers had epileptic children. The higher rate of epileptic offspring when the mother is epileptic may be partially explained by a seizure occurring during pregnancy or other toxic seizure-related factors that may affect a developing fetus.

Stein (1933) found a lower prevalence of epilepsy (2.2%) in 267 offspring of 87 inpatients; nevertheless, this rate was higher than the 0.9% found in the relatives of controls. Because Stein restricted the population he studied to in-patients in a chronic care institution for epileptic patients, and usually obtained family histories from the admission history of the patient or from an occasional follow-up by a social worker, the rate he reported may be unreliably low.

A careful evaluation by Conrad (1937) showed that 6.0% of the offspring of patients with idiopathic epilepsy, 2.7% of the offspring of patients with mixed epilepsy, and 1.6% of the offspring of patients with symptomatic epilepsy had seizures. These rates may not be completely accurate either, because some of the offspring were not definitely epileptic (Harvald, 1954).

Annegers et al. (1976) recently examined the seizure rates in the offspring of epileptic patients in Minnesota. Of 830 live births from 406 epileptic parents, 42 offspring had seizure disorders, and of 826 live births from control parents, only 30 offspring had seizure disorders. The contrast between the seizure rate in offspring of epileptic patients and the expected number of cases in the normal population was greatest between the older offspring of the two groups; therefore, the significance may become greater as the series is followed further. The increased seizure rate of offspring in this study was present only in the offspring born to epileptic mothers, who had approximately five times the normal number of children afflicted with a seizure disorder. Although the increased seizure incidence of the offspring of epileptic mothers could not be correlated with the maternal use of antiepileptic medication or with a seizure during pregnancy, the number of affected offspring was quite small and this lack of correlation might be due to the small numbers studied.

One of the most recent studies was conducted by Tsuboi and Endo (1977), who investigated 506 offspring of epileptic patients and found— similar to the finding of the Annegers study—that the offspring of epileptic mothers had a higher rate of seizures (2.9%) than did the offspring of epileptic fathers (1.7%). If febrile convulsions are also included, considerably higher seizure rates of 11.0% and 6.9% are found for the offspring of epileptic mothers and epileptic fathers, respectively. A control study was not performed.

Judging by these results, the rate of epilepsy of the offspring of unselected epileptic patients is usually higher than in the general population. The offspring rate of epilepsy reaches 10% if all types of seizure are included.

Sibling data. The rate of occurrence of epilepsy in siblings of epileptic patients has also been extensively investigated. In addition to many of the problems already mentioned that make obtaining an accurate sample difficult, the order of birth in a family may also be an important variable (Malzburg, 1973). The older children in a family may have a higher epilepsy rate than younger ones; thus, a small family with few siblings may have a higher seizure rate than a large one.

Stein (1933) investigated the rate of seizures in siblings of 1,000 institutionalized epileptic patients and discovered that of the 945 patients with histories involving siblings, 176 (4.1%) of the 4,305 siblings or half-siblings had a history of epilepsy, as opposed to 35 (0.8%) of the 4,381 siblings of controls. When Paskind and Brown (1937) compared the siblings of institutional patients with siblings of outpatients, they found approximately equal rates: 5.4% of the siblings of the institutional patients had seizures, and 6.6% of the siblings of outpatients had them. Alstrom (1950) calculated that 1.7% of the siblings of unselected epileptic patients had a seizure disorder, but his study did not include the effect of age, a factor that others have found to be significant. An investigation of the siblings of adult patients may indicate a deceptively low seizure rate because an early convulsive history has been lost. Harvald's study (1954) showed that 4.3% of 218 brothers and 2.1% of 207 sisters of epileptic patients also had seizures, but again an analysis according to age was not one of the parameters included.

When epileptic children and their siblings are analyzed, the seizure rates of the siblings are usually higher than expected. Metrakos and Metrakos (1961a), in a study involving primarily children, found that 9.6% of the siblings of epileptic probands had a history of convulsions. Another study by Metrakos (1961) that was limited to probands having centrencephalic and atypical centrencephalic electroencephalograms uncovered the fact that approximately 13% of the siblings of epileptic probands had a seizure history. Van den Berg (1974), when investigating children with febrile convulsions, found that their siblings had a significantly higher rate of febrile convulsions but a nonsignificantly higher rate of nonfebrile convulsions.

Thus, a slight increase in seizure rates has been found in siblings from a large, nonselected seizure population. The prevalence of seizures in siblings is significantly greater than that in siblings of a nonselected seizure population if the probands are restricted to specific seizure types or age groups, of which we shall have more to say later in this review. When all seizure types are included, the rate of epilepsy in siblings approaches 5% and may be higher if the proband has a generalized seizure disorder. That the seizure rate of siblings is lower than the seizure rate of offspring may be explained by several factors, including less complete histories of offspring, the increased age of siblings in these studies as opposed to that of offspring, and, usually, the absence of the nongenetic risk of epilepsy incurred when the mother has epilepsy.

Parental data. The seizure rate of parents of epileptic patients is generally lower than that of siblings or offspring. Stein (1933) reported a rate of 3.5% in 1,000 mothers of epileptics investigated and a rate of 2.3% in 1,000 fathers of epileptics. This slight increase of seizures in women is consistent with the results of other studies and may be related to hormonal influences or other factors already discussed.

Alstrom (1950) reported that 1.7% of the parents of patients having epilepsy with an unknown etiology and 1.2% of the parents of patients having epilepsy with a known etiology had experienced at least one seizure. In a large series Harvald (1951) reported that the mothers of patients with idiopathic epilepsy had a slightly higher prevalence of epilepsy (3.2%) than did the fathers (2.8%), but that parents of idiopathic seizure patients did not have a significantly higher seizure rate than the controls did.

Metrakos and Metrakos (1960) found that 13% of the mothers of epileptics and 5.9% of the fathers of epileptics had a seizure history, compared with 3.8% of the mothers and 0.8% of the fathers in control groups. 11.7% of the parents of the patients with typical centrencephalic electroencephalogram records and 14.6% of the parents of patients with atypical ones had suffered convulsions, compared with 1.34% of the control parents (Metrakos and Metrakos, 1961a).

The higher rates of parental epilepsy in the Metrakos' studies may be partially explained by the young proband population and possibly also by the seizure type of the proband. Although the seizure type was not specifically mentioned by the Metrakos', many patients probably had generalized seizure disorders, judging from the generalized electroencephalogram abnormalities recorded. The seizure rate of the parents of mixed seizure probands is not accurately known, but it is probably between 3 and 10%.

Combinations of Relatives

Most evaluations on the genetics of epilepsy have come from studies of unselected combinations of the relatives of unselected seizure patients. Metrakos and Metrakos (1960) analyzed the seizure rates of the more distant relatives of patients with seizures and found that aunts and uncles had a rate of convulsions of 5.8%, which was somewhat lower than that of parents or siblings; grandparents and cousins had a still lower rate of approximately 1.5% each. Part of this decline from the near-relative rate is probably a result of the methodology applied in the studies, since the rate of epilepsy in control population declined also, with the seizure rate of control siblings being higher than that of aunts or uncles, whose rates were in turn higher than those of grandparents or cousins. Although the data might suggest that epilepsy rates decline in relatives more distant from the proband, this tendency is not proved.

Lumping together a large number of assorted relatives has been a typical method used in many investigations. Researchers such as Gowers (1881), Thom (1915), Lennox and Davis (1950), Tanaka and Aramitsu (1967), Beaussart and Loiseau (1969), Sallou and Poissonnier (1969), Sorel (1969), Soulayrol et al. (1969), Pedersen and Krogh (1971), and Beteta (1972) considered only the percentage of epileptic patients who had a positive family history for epilepsy and not the rates of specific relative groups. Because of the varying methods used to assess epileptic trends in families, the varying sizes of the families themselves, and the omission on the part of the investigators to specify the type of seizure being studied in the probands and their relatives, the percentage of positive family histories has varied from a low of 2.5% (Beaussart and Loiseau, 1969) to a high of between 35 and 50% (Gowers, 1881; Beteta, 1973), with other data found scattered in between these values.

In an attempt to organize the data better, some researchers have subdivided the probands into more specific groups. The relation between age and time of onset of seizures in the proband has been investigated by several groups of researchers, including Soulayrol et al. (1969) and Pedersen and Krogh (1971), who found little correlation between familial seizure rates and the age of onset in the proband. However, Alstrom (1952) found the highest number of positive family histories in children whose seizures had begun before the age of 5.

The effect of proband gender on the familial seizure rate has been investigated by Pedersen and Krogh (1971) and by several earlier workers (Echeverria, 1880; Gowers, 1881; Muskins, 1928), but in most cases proband gender has not significantly affected the familial seizure rate.

However, the type of epilepsy found in the proband is an important factor in the family history, and we shall discuss it more extensively later on in this review. As previously stated, Sorel (1969) found that the prevalence of a familial history of epilepsy in 202 patients who had an idiopathic generalized seizure disorder was 27%, but he also discovered that of 2,488 patients experiencing other types of seizure 1% had a familial history of epilepsy. Tanaka and Aramitsu (1967) found that epileptic patients whose physical examinations were normal had almost twice the number of positive family histories as did those whose examinations were abnormal. If epileptics having generalized epilepsy in addition to a normal neurological examination are specified, an even higher percentage that have positive family histories is found (30–40%).

In addition to studying the percentage of probands with positive family histories, several investigators have based their calculations on a more precise and valuable measurement: the specific seizure rate of collected relatives. Because of the mixed seizure types of patients, the varying closeness of the relative and the difficulties attendant in obtaining accurate histories, these data have varied from lows of 2.7% (Lennox, 1947) and 2.1% (Cobb, 1932) to a high of approximately 15% (Echeverria, 1880).

Several investigators subdivided epileptics into more specific groups. Lennox (1947a) selected patients according to the age of onset of the seizure disorder and found that when the proband's seizures had begun before the age of 4, the seizure rate of relatives was 4.5%; but when the proband's seizures began after the age of 20, the seizure rate of relatives was 1.2%. Eisner et al. (1959) examined the relatives of probands with generalized tonic-clonic seizures who also suffered from an additional seizure disorder and found no significant change from the 4 to 6% seizure rate of the relatives of probands with only generalized tonic-clonic seizures. Cobb (1932) described a low seizure rate of 2.1% in relatives of epilepsy patients, which, nevertheless, was significantly higher than that found in control patients (0–26%). If patients whose epilepsy appears to be secondary to head trauma are analyzed, the seizure rate of their relatives drops to a rate of 1.4%, which is still higher than that of controls. In the series by Harvald (1954) close relatives of idiopathic seizure patients had seizure rates of 3.5% and distant relatives had rates of 2.3%, whereas only one individual of 310 relatives of symptomatic patients had a seizure history.

Thus, studies of familial epilepsy that have involved seizure patients have often yielded mixed results. In the most specific studies an increased seizure frequency is found in the closest and youngest family members. Overall, up to 20% of the epileptic patients have a family member with a seizure history and approximately 5% of their close relatives (siblings, offspring, parents) have suffered a convulsion.

Studies of Probands with a Specific Seizure Type

Generalized Tonic-Clonic Seizures

Eisner et al. (1959, 1960) and Tsuboi and Endo (1977) conducted large studies of probands with generalized tonic-clonic seizures (Table 6). Tsuboi and Endo restricted their study to the offspring of 130 patients who experienced generalized tonic-clonic seizures either with or without an aura. The prevalence of either epileptic attacks or febrile convulsions in the 433 offspring was 9.2%, with a prevalence of seizures alone of 2.3%. Since almost half of the offspring were under the age of 10, however, these rates may rise after later testing. When patients who experienced generalized tonic-clonic seizures without an aura were examined separately, 16.8% of their offspring had either febrile convulsions or seizures and 4.7% of the offspring had seizures alone.

Eisner et al. (1959) found similar trends after examining close relatives (that is, siblings or parents) of epileptic patients. Relatives of idiopathic seizure patients had a seizure rate of 5.26%, which was considerably higher than the control rate of 1.75%. More specifically, those probands whose generalized tonic-clonic seizures had begun before the age of 4 had relatives with the highest epilepsy rates: 8.3%, compared to 1.45% in the control group.

A significant rate of epilepsy is found in the relatives of patients having tonic-clonic seizures when the results of a number of studies

TABLE 6. *Clinical investigations—generalized tonic-clonic seizures*

Investigator	Probands					Relatives			
	Seizure type	No.	Sex	Age range	Relationship	No.	Seizure type	Percent affected
Eisner et al., 1959	Generalized tonic-clonic	136		0–3	Close	662	Generalized tonic-clonic	8.3
	Generalized tonic-clonic	85		4–9		390	Generalized tonic-clonic	4.3
	Generalized tonic-clonic	66		10–15		382	Generalized tonic-clonic	5.8
	Generalized tonic-clonic	34		>16		<64	Generalized tonic-clonic	3.4
Tsuboi and Endo, 1977	Generalized tonic-clonic, alone or mixed	108 122	M F		Offspring Offspring	206 227	Seizure disorder Seizure disorder	7.3 11.0
	Total	230			Offspring	433	Seizure disorder	9.2

on tonic-clonic seizures are combined. Afebrile seizures are found in 7 to 10% of the relatives, and a larger percentage have febrile seizures. This rate, which is considerably higher than that found in the relatives of mixed-seizure patients, reflects the finding that generalized seizures without a known etiology have the strongest genetic tendency.

Absence Attacks

Absence attacks have also been suspected of having a genetic etiology (Table 7). Eisner et al. (1959) found an insignificant increase of epilepsy in the relatives of absence patients, but his group based their study on patients having convulsions and so they did not count absence attacks specifically. Conversely, Matthes and Weber (1968) and Matthes (1969) frequently found a family history of epilepsy in children with absence attacks. A significant number of probands who had absence attacks (13.3%) also had a family history of epilepsy involving either the siblings or parents: 3.1% of the parents had epilepsy, and another 2.3% of the parents had experienced occasional childhood convulsions. The rate of seizures was even higher in siblings, with epilepsy occurring in 3.7% of them and at least an occasional childhood convulsion occurring in another 6.3%. More distant relatives had lower seizure rates, which could have been a result of less accurate histories (a problem mentioned earlier). Doose and Gerken (1972b) found similar results in the siblings of patients with absence attacks and spike-and-wave electroencephalogram discharges. Of the siblings in this study, 6.7% had seizures, the siblings of the female patients having a rate of 9.1%.

The centrencephalic spike-and-wave pattern has also been studied, most notably by Metrakos and Metrakos. This pattern, which is often associated with absence attacks and will be discussed later on in the electroencephalogram section of this review, may be strongly familial.

When the results of the above studies on absence attacks are combined, the seizure rate of the relatives of probands who have absence attacks is significantly higher than normal, with multiple-seizure types represented in the affected relatives. The seizure rate approaches 10% in these probands' relatives and so is comparable to the generalized tonic-

TABLE 7. Absence—clinical investigations

	Probands				Relatives				
Investigator	Seizure description	No.	Sex	Percent with positive family history	Relationship	No.	Sex	Seizure type	Percent affected
Doose and Gerken, 1972b	Absence, spike-wave				Siblings	448 / 200 / 248	M / F	Cerebral seizures	6.7
	Absence, spike-wave		M		Siblings	205 / 92 / 113	M / F	Cerebral seizures	3.9
	Absence spike-wave		F		Siblings	243 / 108 / 135	M / F	Cerebral seizures	9.1
Eisner et al., 1959	Petit mal	34			Close	130		All convulsions / Generalized tonic-clonic	1.37 / 0.66
Jeras and Tividar, 1973	Absence	104 / 64 / 40	F / M	10.6					
Matthes and Weber, 1968	Pyknolepsy	129			Siblings	232		Epilepsy / Absence	3.9 / 3.0

Matthes, 1969	Pyknolepsy	128	Parents	258	Epilepsy	3.1
			Parents	256	Epilepsy	3.1
					Any convulsion	5.4
			Siblings	240	Epilepsy	3.7
					Any convulsion	10.0
			Grandparents, aunts, uncles, and cousins	1,830	Epilepsy	1.3
					Any convulsion	1.7

clonic seizure rate. The seizure rates of the relatives of both absence attack and generalized tonic-clonic epileptics may turn out to be even higher if careful studies are performed on the relatives, including an evaluation of their alertness during the appearance of electroencephalographic abnormalities.

Generalized Seizure Types Other Than Absence and Generalized Tonic-Clonic

Other seizure types have also been associated with an increased familial seizure frequency (Table 8). Lacy and Penry (1976) found that 8 (1.5%) of 548 probands with infantile spasms had a family history of infantile spasms and that 44 (8%) had a family history of epilepsy. Degen (1972), when examining the siblings and parents of patients with infantile spasms, found a history of epilepsy in 10.8% of the families compared to a rate of 2.4% in control children. Since infantile spasms are a collection of disorders that have multiple etiologies, some of which are genetic, the significance of the familial increase is unclear.

The Lennox-Gastaut syndrome, which encompasses a variety of generalized and partial seizure disorders, has been examined by several investigators. Eisner et al. (1959) did not find that myoclonic, akinetic, or atonic seizures were inherited in the patients they studied. Other researchers have found a small but significant correlation between patients with these seizures and inheritance. However, Gastaut et al. (1968) found a family history of epilepsy in 14% of their patients after 25 years of follow-up, and Doose et al. (1970) found a seizure history in the families of 56% of 50 patients who had myoclonic astatic petit mal, with 5.1% of the siblings, parents, and grandparents having a convulsive disorder.

Tsuboi and Christian (1973) investigated relatives of 319 patients with "impulsive petit mal" and discovered that 27.3% of the patients had either a parent, child, or sibling whose history included epilepsy and that 33.5% of the female patients had a positive family history. Again, because of the multiple etiologies of these disorders, the significance of the familial increase to the genetics of epilepsy is unclear.

Other rare seizure types such as familial paroxysmal choreoathetosis (Pryles et al., 1952; Hudgins and Corbin, 1966), kinesthetic reflex epilepsy (Hamaguchi et al., 1969), and photosensitive epilepsy (mentioned by many investigators) have been associated with the familial trend that characterizes other generalized seizures, including generalized tonic-clonic seizures and absence attacks. The etiology of many of these generalized seizure dosorders is not known, although the precipitating event for each type of seizure is known.

Partial Seizures

Investigations have shown that epileptics who have partial seizures have a family history of epilepsy less frequently than epileptics who have generalized seizures (Table 9). Of patients who have partial seizures, the percentage with a positive family history of seizures varies from 1% (Beaussart and Loiseau, 1969) to over 50% (Holowach et al., 1961), the median being approximately 10 to 20% (Rossini et al., 1958; Holowach et al., 1961). These values are obtained if the study is restricted to siblings, parents, and offspring. However, lower values in the close relatives have been found by Penfield and Paine (1955). The wide range of the rate of inheritance of seizures may be explained by the different ages of probands and relatives, different seizure types, and etiologies for the seizures, as well as by the questionable accuracy of some of the family histories, and other variables already mentioned. Comparison with appropriate controls has rarely been done.

Other reports of seizure rates in relatives have been only slightly more consistent, ranging from 1% (Penfield and Paine, 1955) to approximately 10% (Ounstead et al., 1966). Muller et al. (1973) found a seizure rate of 3.2% in 275 parients and 200 siblings of children with partial seizures and a rate of 2.1% in the parents and siblings of controls. Ounstead et al. (1966) conducted a large study of complex partial seizure patients and found a 15% seizure rate in their siblings and an even higher rate when the siblings were of probands who suffered status epilepticus (30%). In this study, febrile seizures occurred quite frequently in probands and relatives, and the episodes of status epilepticus

TABLE 8. *Miscellaneous seizure types*

	Probands					Relatives				
Investigator	Seizure type	No.	Sex	Age range	Percent with positive family history	Relation-ship	No.	Sex	Seizure type	Percent affected
Degen, 1972	Infantile spasms	65			10.8	Siblings	66		"Epileptic"	4.5
Doose et al., 1970	Myoclonic-astatic-petit mal	50			56.0	Parents	128		"Epileptic"	3.1
		35	M			*Total*	194		"Epileptic"	3.6
		15	F			All relatives	602		Convulsions	5.1
							284	M	Convulsions	4.3
							318	F	Convulsions	5.3
						Siblings	95		Convulsions	12.6
						Parents	98		Convulsions	7.1
						Paternal siblings	113		Convulsions	4.4
						Maternal siblings	112		Convulsions	3.6
						Grandparents	184		Convulsions	1.6
Eisner et al., 1959	Minor motor	31				Close	120		Generalized tonic-clonic	0.42
									Convulsions, any type	1.22

Study	Type	n	Age	%	Relationship	n		Seizure	%
Gastaut et al., 1968	Atypical petit mal			14.0					
Matthes, 1969	Myoclonic-astatic	80			Parents	160		Epilepsy	3.1
								Any convulsion	5.1
					Siblings	131		Epilepsy	3.8
								Any convulsion	6.8
Millichap et al., 1962	Infantile spasms	61	0–4 yrs	15.0					
Tsuboi and Christian, 1973	Impulsive petit mal	319	1–54 yrs	27.3	Mixed	1,618		Epilepsy	5.0
						840	M	Epilepsy	3.6
						778	F	Epilepsy	6.5
		161 M	1–54 yrs	21.1	Mixed	787		Epilepsy	2.5
		158 F		33.5	Mixed	831		Epilepsy	7.4
	Impulsive petit mal				Parents	638		Epilepsy	3.3
					Siblings	705		Epilepsy	5.4
					Offspring			Epilepsy	13.6
Zesnov and Erak, 1972	Petit mal variant	32	Children	31.0					

TABLE 9. *Partial seizures*

Investigator	Seizure type	Probands			Percent with positive family history	Relatives					
		No.	Sex	Age range		Relationship	No.	Sex		Seizure type	Percent affected
Andermann, 1972	Focal, treated with surgery	60			71.7	Siblings, parents, offspring	337			Any seizure	3.5
										Epilepsy	1.3
							183	F		Seizure	3.3
										Epilepsy	2.2
							194	M		Seizure	3.6
										Epilepsy	0.5
						Parents	120	60 F		Seizure	0.8
								60 M		Epilepsy	0.8
						Siblings	229	108 F		Seizure	4.8
								121 M		Epilepsy	1.3
						Offspring	28	13 M		Seizure	3.6
								15 F		Epilepsy	3.6
						Grandparents	236			Any seizure	1.3
						Aunts and uncles	737			Any seizure	3.5
						Nieces and nephews	241			Any seizure	1.7
						First cousins	1,608			Any seizure	0.9
Beaussart and Loiseau, 1969	Partial	1,040			1.1						
	Complex partial	780			1.0						
Bray, 1962	Complex partial	15		Children	60.0						
Currie et al., 1971	Complex partial	666	M 316	1–45 yrs	11.0						
			F 350								

Study	Seizure type	N	Age	%	Relationship	N	Outcome	%
Gerken et al., 1977	Mixed and focal EEG abnormalities	198	Children	23.0				
Gerken et al., 1977	Partial seizure with focal EEG				Siblings	157	Seizure	1.9
					Parents	157		3.2
					Father's siblings	181		1.1
					Mother's siblings	230		2.2
					Grandparents	156		1.3
Eisner et al., 1959	Complex partial	11			Close	61	Generalized tonic-clonic	0.0
	Focal	89			Close	466	Convulsion, any type	2.17
								2.7
Holowach et al., 1958	Complex partial	100	11–15 yrs	55.0	All			
				23.0	Parents and siblings			
Holowach et al., 1958	Elementary partial complex	95	1–15 yrs	28.0	All			
				14.0	Parents and siblings			
Jensen, 1975	Complex partial	74		30.0	Siblings	171	Epilepsy	2.9
							Any convulsive disorder	4.7
Lindsay, 1971	Complex partial	99	0–16		Siblings	214	Seizure	15.0
	Complex partial and previous status epilepticus	32			Siblings	76	Seizure	30.0
	Complex partial with cerebral insult	34			Siblings	52	Seizure	1.9

TABLE 9. *(Continued)*

Investigator	Probands Seizure type	No.	Sex	Age range	Percent with positive family history	Relationship	No.	Sex	Seizure type	Percent affected
	Complex partial without status or insult	33				Siblings	86		Seizure	9.0
Muller et al., 1973	Focal	151		Children		Siblings	200		Epilepsy Any convulsive disorder	3.5
						Parents	275		Epilepsy Any convulsive disorder	3.0 3.8
Penfield and Paine, 1955	Focal with temporal lobe surgery	234 153 81	M F		4.4	Near relatives				<1.0
Rossini et al., 1956	Complex partial	100		1–16	10.0					
Shu, 1975	Rolandic epilepsy	158		3–9	24.7					
Tsuboi and Endo, 1977	Complex partial	24 9 15	 M F			Offspring	56		Seizure disorder	8.9
	Focal	9 4 5	 M F			Offspring	17		Seizure disorder	5.9

were usually associated with fever. This association of febrile seizures, heredity and complex partial seizures may be important, because in another study seizures increased considerably (Falconer, 1971) when the proband sample contained a large number of individuals who had prolonged febrile convulsions in childhood.

Andermann (1972) has conducted the most complete genetic study of complex partial seizures. Although she identified several families in which a seizure disorder appeared as either an autosomal dominant or as a recessive pattern, the prevalence of epilepsy in close relatives (1.3%) and of other disorders characterized by at least one seizure (3.5%) was only slightly higher than the control rate of 2.9%, with the highest incidence found in the siblings and the offspring of both probands and controls. As for distant relatives, the seizure rates of nephews and nieces were again higher in the proband group than in the control group, with rates of 2.7% compared with 0.13%. The seizure rate in the control group, however, was extremely low, which raises a question as to the accuracy of the observations. Thus, in most studies of proband populations that consist of patients with partial seizures, 2 to 3% of the relatives have a seizure history, a rate that is only slightly higher than that of controls.

Several investigators have examined other focal seizures in addition to complex partial seizures. A comparison study of the relatives of patients having elementary partial seizures with the relatives of control children who were obtained from several chronic clinic populations (Eisner et al., 1959) showed that the close relatives of the focal patients had a seizure rate of approximately 2.5%, which was indistinguishable from that of the control population but was somewhat greater than the seizure rate usually found in the general population.

Of 95 children having Jacksonian seizures (Holowach et al., 1958), 28% of their close relatives had a seizure history; however, the percentage of all affected relatives was not determined. In several studies the relatively benign seizure disorder associated with a centrotemporal electroencephalographic focus has also shown evidence of a familial tendency; a positive family history was usually present in 25% of the patients (Blom et al., 1972; Shu, 1975) and may be present even more frequently in small groups (Bray, 1962).

Thus, a tendency toward partial seizures, particularly in children, may be inherited, but the evidence supporting this conclusion is not strong and the genetic influence is considerably less than in the case of generalized seizures. Epilepsy associated with centrotemporal spikes and seizures resulting from an antecedent febrile convulsion appear to the most common of the inherited forms of partial seizures, but studies investigating the affected relatives have been few and such conclusions should not be drawn. Currently, apart from centrotemporal spike seizures, no evidence has been found demonstrating a definite genetic etiology of partial seizures.

Febrile Convulsions

We have noted that febrile convulsions have been associated with a positive family history (Table 10). The percentage of patients with febrile convulsions whose family history shows either epilepsy or febrile convulsions has ranged in the larger studies from 10% (Herlitz, 1941) to 40 to 50% (Lennox, 1949; Ounsted, 1966; Frantzen et al., 1970).

Millichap (1968) summarized the literature on febrile convulsions and found that 17% of 2,109 patients with febrile convulsions had a family history of febrile convulsions. After another review of the literature, he obtained the histories of 3,771 patients with febrile convulsions of which 32% had a family history of a convulsion of some type and 15% had a family history of epilepsy. A significant percentage of the relatives in both reviews had a history of either febrile convulsions or epilepsy.

Frantzen et al. (1970) studied a series of 2,908 children with febrile convulsions and discovered that 8.2% of the parents had a history of febrile convulsions and another 1.0% had a history of epilepsy. Of the siblings, 10.9% had febrile convulsions and another 0.7% had epilepsy. Most other studies also indicate seizure rates in close relatives of about 10% (Herlitz, 1941; Lennox-Buchthal, 1971; Schiottz-Christensen, 1972; Mollica et al., 1973; van den Berg, 1974), although occasionally slightly higher figures are seen (Ounsted et al., 1966).

In a study of 570 siblings of approximately 1,000 probands, 25.3%

TABLE 10. *Febrile convulsions—clinical investigations*

Investigator	Proband					Relatives			
	Epilepsy type	No.	Sex	Age range	Percent with positive family history	Relationship	No.	Seizure description	Percent affected
Frantzen et al., 1969	Febrile convulsions	194			50.0 18.0			Convulsion, any type Epilepsy	
Frantzen et al., 1970	Febrile convulsions	208			50.0 40.0 20.0			Convulsion, any type Febrile convulsions Epilepsy	
		208				Parents Siblings	146 303	Febrile convulsions	8.2 10.9
Graveleau, 1974	Febrile convulsions	667			21.0				
Herlitz, 1941	Febrile convulsions	420			9.5	Parents Siblings	615	Febrile convulsions or epilepsy	12.4
	Febrile convulsions with a negative family history of parents	380							
	Febrile convulsions with a positive family history of parents	34				Siblings	44	Febrile convulsions or epilepsy	15.9
Hrbek, 1957	Febrile convulsions (hospitalized)	274	(55% M) (45% F)	0–14	31.0	All			
Kagawa, 1975	Febrile convulsions	307				Siblings		Febrile convulsions	19.86

TABLE 10. *(Continued)*

Investigator	Proband						Relatives			
	Epilepsy type	No.	Sex		Age range	Percent with positive family history	Relation-ship	No.	Seizure description	Percent affected
Lennox, 1949	Febrile convulsions					50.0				
Lupu et al. 1971	Febrile convulsions	86				17.0				
Metrakos and Metrakos, 1960	Simple febrile convulsions	88					Parents	176	Febrile convulsions Afebrile convulsions	13.6 3.4
							Siblings	215	Febrile convulsions Afebrile convulsions	9.8 4.7
Millicap et al., 1960	Febrile convulsions	95				30.0				
Mollica et al., 1973	Febrile convulsions	109 57 52	M F		Children	46.0				
Ounstead et al., 1966	Febrile convulsions				Children		Siblings	570	Convulsive disorder Febrile convulsion Epilepsy	25.3 17.9 9.7
	Febrile convulsions with meningitis				Children		Siblings	108	Convulsive disorder Febrile convulsion Epilepsy	6.4 5.5 1.8
	Febrile convulsion followed by remittant epilepsy				Children		Siblings	116	Convulsive disorder Febrile convulsion Epilepsy	17.0 12.0 5.0

Study	N	Condition	Age		Relatives	Outcome	%
		Febrile convulsion followed by chronic epilepsy	Children		Siblings	75 Convulsive disorder	7.0
						Febrile convulsion	4.0
						Epilepsy	3.0
		Febrile convulsions with death	Children		Siblings	58 Convulsive disorder	30.0
						Febrile convulsion	17.0
						Epilepsy	17.0
Ounstead, 1966	100	Febrile convulsions	Children	41.0			
Schiottz-Christensen, 1972	64	Febrile convulsions	6–21		Siblings	Febrile convulsions	14.0
Van den Berg, 1974	144	Febrile convulsions			Siblings (older)	323 Convulsions	11.5
	98				Siblings (younger)	109 Convulsions	9.2

of the siblings had a convulsive disorder, with 17.9% having febrile convulsions, and 9.7% having epilepsy (Ounsted et al., 1966). This study, although it is convincing because of its large size, lacked controls and included relatively few siblings per proband. The relatives of the probands whose febrile convulsions resulted in death had the highest seizure rate (30%) of convulsions of any type. The most recent studies (the NINCDS collaborative perinatal project) show that 7.6% of close relatives have a history of only febrile convulsions (Nelson and Ellenberg, 1978). Thus, febrile convulsions are associated with a strong family history of both febrile and afebrile convulsions.

Of several pedigree patterns that have been associated with febrile convulsions, an autosomal dominant pattern is the most common (Lennox-Buchthal, 1973), but evidence from twin studies indicates that a polygenetic mechanism may also be involved. However, the pattern of inheritance remains uncertain because of the lack of control studies. Indeed, the inheritance pattern may vary from family to family.

Seizures with a Known Etiology

Seizures secondary to a known cause (symptomatic seizures) have not shown as strong a hereditary pattern as idiopathic seizures have (Table 11). Several investigators have reported a seizure rate of approximately 1.5% in close relatives (Cobb, 1932; Conrad, 1937; Lennox, 1947a; Eisner et al., 1959), although higher rates have occasionally been reported (Smith et al., 1954). Nearly all of these studies did not include control groups.

Hemiplegic or hemiparetic children with seizures have a significantly higher percentage of relatives with seizures than do hemiplegic children who are free of seizures (Rimoin and Metrakos, 1963). Convulsions associated with smallpox vaccinations indicate a familial pattern, and frequently when a history of seizures of electroencephalographic abnormalities is found in a patient, a history of seizures is also found in near relatives (Doose et al., 1968). An association between a family history of epilepsy and convulsions during pregnancy in previously non-epileptic individuals has been observed (Rosenbaum and Maltby, 1943;

TABLE 11. Seizures with a known etiology

| Investigator | Proband | | | | | Relatives | | | | | |
	Seizure type or cause	No.	Sex	Age range	Percent with positive family history	No.	Sex	Age range	Relation-ship	Seizure description	Percent affected
Cobb, 1932	Head trauma	235									1.4
Conrad, 1937	Symptomatic epilepsy	54 25	M F	35–90		275 130 145	M F	0–64	Offspring	Epilepsy	1.62
Eisner et al., 1959	"Organic"	83				469			Close	All types Generalized tonic-clonic Other	2.2 1.8 0.4
Doose et al., 1968	Smallpox vaccination	171 87 84	M F	Children	58.0						
Harvald, 1951	"Symptomatic"					680 661 242 248	M F M F		Siblings Siblings Parents Parents	Epilepsy Epilepsy Epilepsy Epilepsy	1.46 0.95 0.86 0.0
Harvald, 1954	"Symptomatic"					123 197 320			Close Distant All	Epilepsy Epilepsy Epilepsy	1.0 0.0 0.3
Lennox, 1947	"Symptomatic"					2,714					

TABLE 11. *(Continued)*

| Investigator | Proband | | | | | Relatives | | | | | |
	Seizure type or cause	No.	Sex	Age range	Percent with positive family history	No.	Sex	Age range	Relation- ship	Seizure description	Percent affected
Lennox, 1951	"Symptomatic"			All		4,310			Near	Epilepsy	1.8
				0–1		1,023				Epilepsy	2.9
				2–4		562				Epilepsy	2.0
				5–9		759				Epilepsy	1.4
				10–19		831				Epilepsy	1.4
				20–29		451				Epilepsy	1.1
				>30		684				Epilepsy	1.3
Lindsay, 1971	Complex partial seizures with cerebral insult	34		0–16		52			Siblings	Seizures	1.9
MacIntosh, 1952	Eclampsia	21	F		30.0						
Meyer, 1976	Ethanol withdrawal	55				309			Close		1.3
Pedersen, 1964	Postencephalitic	33			12.1						
Rimon and Metrakos, 1963	Convulsive disorder and hemiplegia	98		Children		3,776			Near relatives	Seizure disorder	2.04
						192			Parents	Seizure disorder	2.6
						231			Siblings	Seizure disorder	5.6

Study	Condition	N	Sex		Relationship	N		Rate
Rosenbaum et al., 1943	Eclampsia	20	F					60.0
	Preclampsia	20	F					10.0
Smith et al., 1954	Acquired epilepsy	535		Average 5–9	Aunts and uncles Grandparents	1,076	Seizure disorder	24.0 / 3.9
						384	Seizure disorder	1.8
Tanaka and Aramitsu, 1962	Patients with neurological deficit	64			Cousins	1,899	Seizure disorder	0.5
		37	M					6.9
		27	F					

MacIntosh, 1952). Epilepsy secondary to supratentorial astrocytomas may have a familial tendency also (Lund, 1952). Pedersen (1964) noted four patients who had a family history of epilepsy from a total of 33 patients whose epilepsy was secondary to encephalitis; one had a convulsion after a smallpox vaccination, and the other three were infants. Epilepsy associated with alcohol abuse has not shown a significant genetic tendency (Giove, 1965; Meyer et al., 1976), but the studies on it have been small. Epilepsy occurring with renal insufficiency and hemodialysis has been associated with a positive family history (Gastaut et al., 1971).

The relation between posttraumatic epilepsy and genetics is controversial (Pampus and Seidenfaden, 1974). When 739 men who had sustained head injuries in World War II were investigated, a slightly but not significantly higher prevalence of familial epilepsy was found in patients who developed seizures compared with those who did not (Walker, 1962). A family history of epilepsy was reported in 7% of 80 posttraumatic seizure patients as opposed to only 2% of those who did not develop seizures (Evans, 1962). Possibly posttraumatic seizures are secondary to a genetic factor that causes exaggerated hypertrophic scars and keloid formation (Hioppner et al., 1973).

Whether a genetic trend exists in symptomatic seizure patients remains controversial. Most studies have suggested a slight increase in positive family histories of these seizure patients, but few well-controlled studies exist. If a genetic trend is present, it is not prominent.

ELECTROENCEPHALOGRAPHIC STUDIES

Numerous investigators have used electroencephalograms to study the genetics of epilepsy, as mentioned in reviews of the subject by Doose and Gerken, 1972a; Degen, 1975. Electroencephalographic studies have been done on the pedigrees of epileptics, on twins, and on the relatives of large groups of probands. In most studies electroencephalographic abnormalities, either generalized or focal, are more frequently present in the relatives than an actual seizure history is. However, a significant percentage of nonepileptic individuals may also have these electroencephalographic abnormalities. Apparently, such abnormalities are not confined to epileptics.

Multiple Seizure Types and Mixed Electroencephalographic Abnormalities in Relatives

Several investigators have studied the electroencephalograms of relatives who have multiple seizure types (Table 12). They found that the abnormality rate of the relatives' electroencephalograms is about 30%, depending on the criteria set for abnormality and the type of patients selected. Early investigators such as Lennox et al. (1939, 1940) found electroencephalographic abnormalities in over 50% of the close relatives of epileptics; however, spike-and-wave discharges were considerably less frequent in the close relatives (less than 10%), whose abnormalities consisted mostly of either abundant fast activity or excessive slow waves.

Similar trends have been found more recently (Richter, 1956; Kishimoto et al., 1961; Znamierowaska-Kozik, 1964; Petrischenko, 1968; Lipinski et al., 1975). Electroencephalographic abnormalities have been reported in 30 to 40% of the close relatives of epileptics. Most of the changes consisted of background abnormalities or paroxysmal rhythm disturbances without definite spikes; spike activity only appeared in approximately 10 to 15% of the abnormal electroencephalograms of close relatives. However, the specificity of these findings is doubtful because the electroencephalographic abnormalities have usually not been correlated with clinical and historical examinations of the relatives.

Generalized Seizure Types and Generalized Electroencephalographic Abnormalities in Relatives

Several investigators have studied the electroencephalograms of relatives of patients having either generalized seizures or generalized electroencephalogram abnormalities. The photoconvulsive responses and the photic-induced seizures, which logically should be mentioned here are discussed extensively in another review (Newmark and Penry, 1979). Rodin and Gonzalez (1966) examined the relatives of 20 patients with

TABLE 12. Multiple seizure types—EEG studies

	Probands						Relatives				
Investigator	EEG or epilepsy type	No.	Sex	Age range	Percent with positive family history	Relation-ship	No.	Sex	Age range	EEG pattern	Percent affected
Beteta, 1972	Convulsive disorder	100		0–3 yr	40.0						
Harvald, 1954	Mixed with markedly abnormal EEG					Near	145	M		Slightly abnormal	21.4
										Markedly abnormal	10.3
										Focal	0.7
							147	F		Slightly abnormal	36.7
										Markedly abnormal	18.4
										Focal	0.7
						Distant	114	M		Slightly abnormal	14.9
										Markedly abnormal	7.0
							104	F		Slightly abnormal	41.3
										Markedly abnormal	10.6
										Focal	1.0
	Mixed with normal or slightly abnormal EEG					Near	69	M		Slightly abnormal	29.0
										Markedly abnormal	4.3

Study	Diagnosis	n	Sex	Relationship	n	Sex	Age	EEG finding	%
					54	F		Slightly abnormal	40.7
								Markedly abnormal	3.7
				Distant	22	M		Slightly abnormal	13.6
					36	F		Slightly abnormal	36.1
								Markedly abnormal	2.8
Kishimoto et al., 1961	Idiopathic epilepsy	48		Parents, siblings, or offspring	86			Abnormal	50.0
		21	M		44			Abnormal	43.0
		21	F		42			Abnormal	57.0
Lennox et al., 1939	Mixed	76		Mixed parents, offspring, and siblings	138	M		Dysrhythmia	54.0
					100	F			
Lennox et al., 1940	Mixed	94		Parents	61	M	3–78	Abnormal	54.1
					82	F		Abnormal	62.0
				Siblings and offspring	19	M		Abnormal	53.0
					21	F		Abnormal	76.0
				Near	14		0–12	Abnormal	43.0
					8		13–16	Abnormal	100.0
					22		17–29	Abnormal	50.0
					37		30–39	Abnormal	57.0
					54		40–49	Abnormal	59.0
					49		>50	Abnormal	51.0
Lennox et al., 1942	Mixed	149			280			Abnormal	52.0

TABLE 12. (Continued)

| Investigator | Probands | | | | Percent with positive family history | Relatives | | | | | EEG pattern | Percent affected |
	EEG or epilepsy type	No.	Sex	Age range		Relation-ship	No.	Sex	Age range			
Lipinski et al., 1975	Mixed	275				Offspring	282		3–11		Generalized spike-wave	14.4
						Negative neurolog-ical history	125		3–11		Generalized spike-wave	14.4
						Positive neurolog-ical history	150		3–11		Generalized spike-wave	14.6
Petrischenko, 1968	Mixed	35					70				Paroxysmal discharges	51.0
Rimon and Metrakos, 1965	Mixed con-vulsive dis-orders	98		Children		Parents	34				Epileptiform	15.0
						Siblings	37				Epileptiform	3.0
Richter, 1956	Mixed	43				Parent	23	M			Dysrhythmia	8.7
						Parent	22	F			Dysrhythmia	36.0
						Offspring	6	M			Epileptiform	16.6
						Offspring	5	F			Abnormal	0.0
						Sibling	11	M			Abnormal	18.0
						Sibling	14	F			Dysrhythmia	29.0
Strauss et al., 1939	Mixed	31				Siblings	63				Abnormal	28.6
						Parents	30				Abnormal	23.3
Znamierowska-Kozik, 1964	Mixed	50		4–19		Close	139				Abnormal "Paroxysmal"	32.0 / 10.8

generalized tonic-clonic seizures electroencephalographically and found that 30% of the fathers, 45% of the mothers, and 46% of the siblings had abnormal electroencephalograms consisting of abnormal background rhythms or spike discharges.

When 194 parents of absence probands were examined electroencephalographically (Matthes and Weber, 1968; Matthes, 1969), pathological findings were evident in 34%, with 2.5% having 3/sec spike-and-wave activity and 6.2% having other epileptiform discharges. Of the siblings, 39% had an abnormal electroencephalogram, with 9.2% having 3/sec spike-and-wave activity and 3.7% having other spike discharges. Age was not specifically mentioned, although the younger relatives of the siblings had a significantly higher rate of abnormality than the older ones.

Somewhat conflicting results were found when the relatives of children having myoclonic astatic attacks were evaluated (Matthes, 1969; Doose et al., 1970; Doose, 1971). Although Matthew found that 22.7% of the siblings had a pathological electroencephalogram, only 2.9% had spike-and-wave discharges and 1.9% had other epileptiform activity. In Doose's reports, however, 45.8% of the siblings had abnormal tracings and 8.3% had spike-and-wave discharges. Age was a significant factor in the patients and siblings collected by Doose, who found the greatest number of abnormalities in siblings under the age of 15.

Many studies on the genetics of epilepsy have been classified according to the probands' electroencephalograms (Metrakos and Metrakos, 1961; Metrakos et al., 1966; Rodin and Gonzalez, 1966; Metrakos and Metrakos, 1969). Most of the studies have been restricted to probands who have a centrencephalic electroencephalogram pattern, which is usually defined as a generalized spike-and-wave (Table 13).

In the studies shown in Table 13 (the Rodin and Gonzalez investigation grouped several abnormalities), a centrencephalic pattern was present in almost 50% of the siblings in a susceptible age group of between 4 and 16 years (Metrakos and Metrakos, 1961). Of the parents, 7.69% had centrencephalographic tracings and 9.32% had manifested electroencephalographic abnormalities. Of the siblings, 36.8% had centrencephalic tracings and over 46% had epileptiform abnormalities. How-

TABLE 13: *Generalized seizure disorders—EEG studies*

	Probands					Relatives				
Investigator	EEG or epilepsy type	No. Sex	Age range	Percent with positive family history	Relationship	No. Sex	Age range	EEG type	Percent affected
Doose et al., 1970b	Centrencephalic Myoclonic-astatic-petit mal	51 36 M 15 F	Children	6.0	Siblings	72		PCR Abnormal rhythms Spike-and-wave Abnormal total	27.8 19.4 8.3 45.8
Doose and Gerken, 1972b	Spike-and-wave absence				Siblings	242 108 M 134 F		Abnormal	27.7
Lennox and Davis, 1950	3/sec spike-and-wave	193		34.2					
Matthes, 1969	Myoclonic-astatic	67		7.5	Siblings Parents	98 129		Pathologic Epileptiform Centrencephalic Epileptiform	22.4 5.1 4.6 1.6
Matthes, and Weber, 1968	3/sec spike-and-wave absence	129			Siblings Parents	164 197		3/sec spike-wave 3/sec spike-wave	9.2 2.5
Metrakos and Metrakos, 1961	Centrencephalic	211 108 F			Parents	195		Centrencephalic Epileptiform	7.69 9.23

Author, year		M			Diagnosis	Relation	n	Age range	EEG finding	%
Metrakos et al., 1966	103	M			Centrencephalic epilepsy	Siblings	223		Centrencephalic Epileptiform total	36.77 46.2
						Parents and siblings	59	0–4.5	Centrencephalic	25.4
							79	4.5–8.5	Centrencephalic	44.3
							49	8.5–12.5	Centrencephalic	44.9
							18	12.5–16.5	Centrencephalic	44.4
							9	16.5–20.5	Centrencephalic	22.2
							17	20.5–24.5	Centrencephalic	11.8
							26	24.5–28.5	Centrencephalic	7.7
							42	28.5–32.5	Centrencephalic	7.1
							44	32.5–36.5	Centrencephalic	11.4
							35	36.5–40.5	Centrencephalic	5.7
							24	40.5–44.5	Centrencephalic	4.2
						Offspring	82	4.75–10.5	Centrencephalic	35.0
							51			51.0
							24	<4.75	Centrencephalic	8.0
							7	>16.5	Centrencephalic	14.0
Metrakos and Metrakos, 1967				½–5 yrs	Febrile convulsions	Siblings	147		Spike and wave Epileptiform	21.0 31.0
Metrakos and Metrakos, 1970	81				Febrile convulsions	Parents	86		Centrencephalic Epileptiform	12.8 28.4
						Siblings	104		Centrencephalic Epileptiform	29.8 24.0
Rodin and Gonzalez, 1966	20		35.0		Generalized tonic-clonic	Fathers			Abnormal	30.0
						Mothers			Abnormal	45.0
						Siblings			Abnormal	46.0
	20		70.0		Generalized sharp waves	Fathers			Abnormal	35.0
						Mothers			Abnormal	56.0
						Siblings			Abnormal	55.0

TABLE 13. *(Continued)*

Investigator	EEG or epilepsy type	No.	Sex	Age range	Percent with positive family history	Relationship	No.	Sex	Age range	EEG type	Percent affected
Tsuboi and Christian, 1973	Impulsive petit mal	136				All	390	M		Epileptiform	15.1
							182	M		Epileptiform	14.3
							208	F		Epileptiform	15.9
						Parents	128			Epileptiform	9.4
						Siblings	128			Epileptiform	13.3
						Offspring	114			Epileptiform	24.6
	Impulsive	65	M			All	185			Epileptiform	12.4
	petit mal	71	F			All	205			Epileptiform	17.6
	Impulsive			0–9 yrs		All	57			Epileptiform	21.0
	petit mal			10–14 yrs		All	144			Epileptiform	10.4
				15–19 yrs		All	163			Epileptiform	16.0
				>20 yrs		All	36			Epileptiform	16.7
Tsuboi and Endo, 1977	"Generalized"	63				Offspring	102			Epileptiform	37.3

ever, the high percentage of abnormalities in controls complicated the specificity of this study: 8.7% had centrencephalic tracings and 15.5% had epileptiform activity in a population that did not have a high seizure rate.

A study of the offspring of epileptic patients revealed generalized spike-and-wave discharges in 14.5%, in contrast to only 1.7% in the offspring of controls (Lipinski, 1975).

Thus, a centrencephalic record is common in close relatives of epileptic patients, particularly those relatives in a susceptible age group between 4 and 16 years, but the specificity of this pattern remains uncertain. Also, reports tracing the highest rates of electroencephalographic abnormalities show that a prominent contrast exists between clinical and electroencephalogram findings. A more specific definition of abnormality may be required before the significance of electroencephalogram abnormalities can be known. Long-term studies of relatives and their offspring should be undertaken to observe the development of seizures, and specific clinical testing should be performed on the electroencephalogram-positive relatives to determine whether an occult seizure disorder exists. In patients with absence attacks, impairment of consciousness is closely correlated with spike-and-wave discharges (Browne et al., 1974), If a similar correlation can be demonstrated in allegedly asymptomatic relatives experiencing spike-and-wave discharges, the significance of the electroencepohalogram findings will be greatly enhanced.

Partial Seizure Types and Focal Electroencephalographic Abnormalities in Relatives

Although the investigation grouped the probands according to seizure type, most studies classified the probands according to the focal abnormalities found on their electroencephalograms (Table 14). In Rodin's and Gonzales' analysis (1966) a significant percentage of the relatives of probands who were diagnosed as having focal sharp waves also had abnormal tracings: 25% of the fathers, 43% of the mothers, and 31% of the siblings. Two difficulties with this study are the broad definition of abnormality that was used and the lack of a control group.

TABLE 14. *Focal probands—EEG studies*

| | Probands | | | | | Relatives | | | | | |
Investigator	EEG or epilepsy type	No.	Sex	Age range	Percent with positive family history	Relation-ship	No.	Sex	Age range	EEG type	Percent affected
Andermann, 1972	Focal, treated by surgery	60			71.7	Close	167		mean 31.3	Abnormal	32.9
										Epileptiform	16.8
							68	M	mean 31.5	Abnormal	25.0
										Epileptiform	10.3
							99	F	mean 31.2	Abnormal	38.4
										Epileptiform	21.2
						Parents	61		mean 52.6	Abnormal	24.6
										Epileptiform	8.2
						Siblings	85		mean 21.3	Abnormal	37.6
							35			Epileptiform	20.0
						Offspring	21		mean 10.3	Abnormal	38.1
										Epileptiform	28.6
						Aunts and uncles	21		mean 45.0	Abnormal	33.3
										Epileptiform	14.3
						Nieces and nephews	69		mean 10.3	Abnormal	56.5
										Epileptiform	31.9
						Grand-parents	2		mean 74.5	Abnormal	50.0
										Epileptiform	0.0
						First cousins	47		mean 13.3	Abnormal	44.7
										Epileptiform	17.0
Andermann and Metrakos, 1969	Focal, treated by surgery	48				All	216		5–9	Abnormal	38.4
										Abnormal	72.0

Blom et al., 1972	Rolandic, centrotemporal spike	40	0–13	40.0	All			Focal centro-temporal spike	36.0
				18.0	Siblings and parents			Focal centro-temporal spike	19.0
Bray and Wiser, 1964	Centrotemporal spike	40		30.0	Siblings and offspring	53			
					Parents	21			
Bray and Wiser, 1965a	Centrotemporal spike	40		30.0	All	14	0–5	Midtemporal spike	14.0
						36	6–10		56.0
						26	11–15		42.0
						10	16–20		30.0
						7	21–25		14.0
						38	26–60		13.0
Bray and Wiser, 1965b	Centrotemporal spikes	40			Siblings and offspring	77		Diffuse spike-wave	13.0
					Parents	31		Diffuse spike-wave	16.0
					Aunts and uncles	20		Diffuse spike-wave	20.0
					Nieces and Nephews	60		Diffuse spike-wave	5.0
					Cousins	58		Diffuse spike-wave	5.0
Doose et al., 1977	Focal spikes and epilepsy	198	Children		Siblings	312, M 152, F 160		Spike-wave	3.0

TABLE 14. *(Continued)*

Investigator	Probands EEG or epilepsy type	No.	Sex	Age range	Percent with positive family history	Relatives Relation-ship	No.	Sex	Age range	EEG type	Percent affected
Harvald, 1954	Mixed seizures					Siblings	85		1–4		1.0
						Siblings	96		5–8		6.0
						Siblings	81		9–12		0.0
						Siblings	50		>12		6.0
						Close	67	M		Slightly abnormal	7.5
							65	F		Slightly abnormal	21.5
										Markedly abnormal	4.6
						Distant	42	M		Slightly abnormal	11.9
							36	F		Slightly abnormal	33.3
										Markedly abnormal	6.3
Heijbel et al., 1975	Centrotemporal spike	19	M	5–16	68.0	Parents	38		½–18	Seizures	11.0
		9	F			Siblings	34			Seizures	15.0
							18	M			
							16	F			
						Siblings	32			Rolandic discharge	34.0

Study	Proband type	N	Relatives	N	Sex	EEG finding	%
Metrakos and Metrakos, 1969	Probands with focal EEG		Siblings	127		Spike and wave	18.0
	Treatment with surgery for epilepsy	48	Siblings	63		Epileptiform	24.0
						Spike and wave	12.0
						Epileptiform	22.0
Rodin and Gonzalez, 1966	Complex partial	20	Parents		M	Abnormal	27.0
		50.0	Parents		F	Abnormal	58.0
			Siblings			Abnormal	33.0
	Focal temporal spikes	20	Parents		M	Abnormal	25.0
		35.0	Parents		F	Abnormal	43.0
			Siblings			Abnormal	31.0

Doose et al. (1977) investigated the siblings of epileptic probands who had demonstrated a focal discharge in at least one electroencephalogram. Three percent of all 312 siblings studied and 8% of the siblings between the ages of 5 and 6 had spike-and-wave discharges at rest, rates that were slightly higher than those of the controls. The siblings also had a higher prevalence of photoconvulsive responses (which were defined as either generalized or occipital paroxysmal spike discharges) than did the controls. Only 2.9% of the siblings had focal sharp waves, a rate not significantly higher than the 1.3% seen in control children. Because many probands exhibited photosensitivity or generalized spike-and-wave discharges at rest in addition to the focal discharges, the slight increase of generalized electrical abnormalities of siblings may not be specific for focal probands but may instead reflect the generalized abnormality present in the probands.

Most of the other investigators of focal discharges have stressed the hereditary aspects of two foci: the anterior temporal spike and the mid-temporal spike. The most careful studies of the focal discharges localized in the anterior temporal lobe were conducted by Andermann (1972) during examinations of the relatives of 60 probands who underwent seizure surgery in Montreal. Of 315 relatives of these patients, 40% had an abnormal electroencephalogram and almost 20% of the relatives had an epileptiform tracing, with 11% (35 relatives) experiencing generalized spike-and-wave discharges, and 12% (47 relatives) having a focal record. At the peak age group of between 5 and 15 years over 50% had an abnormal tracing, and approximately 33% had epileptiform discharges. Abnormal tracings and epileptiform discharges were more common in female relatives, particularly in those of the susceptible age group, 5 to 15 years. The rate of abnormality was highest in close relatives (parents, siblings, and offspring), with almost 33% having an abnormal tracing and about 17% having epileptiform discharges. The specificity of this report, however, is clouded by the high rates of abnormalities found in the relatives of controls; almost 21% had an abnormal electroencephalogram and 12% had epileptiform discharges. A female preponderance was also found in the control relatives. Approximately 3% of the control relatives, 4% of the control siblings, and 5% of the focal proband siblings had suffered seizures. These percentages, which are considerably below the electroencephalographic percentages, emphasize the lack of specificity for epilepsy of the above electroencephalographic data.

The midtemporal, or centrotemporal, spike is the second major type of focal seizure that has been studied. According to a series of studies (Bray and Wiser, 1964, 1965a, 1965b) the focal sharp waves, or spikes, are present in 36% of the siblings and the offspring of the probands and are present in 19% of the parents—rates that are higher than those found in controls. In addition to this focal discharge, 13% of the siblings and the offspring and 16% of the parents had diffuse bilateral abnormalities consisting of either paroxysmal spike, slow wave, or spike and slow wave discharges. These percentages were significantly higher than those of controls. In a similar study by Heijbel et al. (1975), 34% of the siblings but only 3% of the parents had centrotemporal discharges. They concluded that the disorder is age dependent, possibly secondary to an autosomal dominant gene.

Thus, epilepsy patients who had focal discharges in the anterior temporal or in the centrotemporal head regions also had close relatives who demonstrated an increased rate of both focal and generalized electroencephalographic abnormalities. In patients with centrotemporal spikes a genetic tendency toward a specific disorder may well exist. Evidence for a genetic basis of anterior temporal spikes is not as clear because the largest series indicated high positive electroencephalographic rates in the control groups also. As already mentioned, the electroencephalographic evidence would more clearly support a genetic basis, in this case for partial seizures, if future studies demonstrated the development of clinical attacks in affected relatives.

C. TWIN STUDIES

Since the early report by Wilson and Wolfson (1929) of generalized tonic-clonic seizures in monozygotic twins, several investigators have examined the seizure rates in monozygotic and dizygotic twins who had a variety of seizure disorders (Tables 15 and 16). In almost all of

TABLE 15. *Twin studies—clinical*

Investigator	Seizure type	No. of twin pairs	Sex of twin pairs	Zygosity	Age range	Co-twin's seizure type	Concordance
Badalyan et al., 1970	Mixed	15		Monozygotic	1.5–16	Mixed	80.0
		20		Dizygotic	1.5–16	Mixed	5.0
Braconi, 1962	Mixed	20	11 M	Monozygotic		Mixed	80.0
			9 F	Monozygotic			
	Idiopathic			Monozygotic		Mixed	91.0
	Symptomatic			Monozygotic		Mixed	62.5
	Mixed	31	9 M	Dizygotic		Mixed	35.0
			12 F				
			10 Mixed				
	Idiopathic			Dizygotic			50.0
	Symptomatic			Dizygotic			14.5
Catalano, 1974	Absence, GTC	30	F	Monozygotic	6–18	Absence, GTC	100.0
	Absence, GTC	4	F	Dizygotic	10–18	Absence, GTC	100.0
Conrad, 1935	Mixed	30	18 M	Monozygotic		Mixed	66.6
			12 F				
	Idiopathic epilepsy			Monozygotic			86.3
	Acquired epilepsy			Monozygotic			12.5
	Mixed	127		Dizygotic		Mixed	3.1
	Idiopathic			Dizygotic			4.3
	Acquired epilepsy			Dizygotic			0.0
Gedda and Tatarelli, 1977	Essential general-ized attacks	19	10 M	Monozygotic	0–13	Generalized epilepsy	94.7
		26		Dizygotic			15.4

Study	Seizure type	N	Sex	Zygosity	Age range	Seizure type	Concordance
Inouye, 1960	Mixed	15	M	Monozygotic	2–86	Mixed	66.7
	Mixed	11	F	Monozygotic	7–32	Mixed	36.4
	Generalized tonic-clonic	14	M	Dizygotic	5–30		14.3
		6	F	Dizygotic	5–40		0.0
		1	Mixed	Dizygotic	16–23		0.0
Lennox-Buchthal, 1971	Febrile convulsions	19		Monozygotic		Febrile convulsions	68.4
						Febrile convulsions plus nocturnal convulsions	89.5
Lennox, 1947	Mixed without etiology	24		Monozygotic		Mixed	83.0
	Mixed with etiology	19		Monozygotic		Mixed	16.0
	Mixed without etiology	16		Dizygotic		Mixed	6.0
	Mixed with etiology	7		Dizygotic		Mixed	0.0
Lennox, 1951	Mixed without etiology	45		Monozygotic		Seizure disorder	84.0
	Mixed with etiology	24		Monozygotic		Seizure disorder	17.0
	Mixed without etiology	40		Dizygotic		Seizure disorder	10.0
	Mixed with etiology	13		Dizygotic		Seizure disorder	0.8
Rosanoff et al., 1934	Mixed	9	M	Monozygotic		Epilepsy	56.0
		14	F	Monozygotic		Epilepsy	64.0

TABLE 15. *(Continued)*

Investigator	Seizure type	No. of twin pairs	Sex of twin pairs	Zygosity	Age range	Co-twin's seizure type	Concordance
		15	M	Dizygotic		Epilepsy	20.0
		24	F	Dizygotic		Epilepsy	16.7
		45	Mixed	Dizygotic		Epilepsy	28.9
Schiottz-Christensen, 1972a	Febrile	14	M	Monozygotic	6–21	Convulsions	16.7
		12	F	Monozygotic	6–21	Convulsions	58.3
		19	M	Dizygotic	6–21	Convulsions	15.8
		18	F	Dizygotic	6–21	Convulsions	11.1
Vercelletto and Courjon, 1969	Mixed	14		Monozygotic		Mixed	71.0
		4		Dizygotic		Mixed	25.0
Wilson and Wolfsohn, 1929	Convulsion	1	F	Monozygotic	22	Convulsions	100.0

TABLE 16. *Twin studies—EEG studies*

Investigator	EEG or seizure type	No. of twin pairs	Sex of twin pairs	Zygosity	Age range	Second twin's EEG pattern	Concordance
Badalyan et al., 1971	Mixed	7		Monozygotic	1.5–16	Similar	71.0
		9		Dizygotic	1.5–16	Similar	0.0
Little and Weaver, 1950	Mixed	3		Monozygotic	4–24		33.0
			1 M	Monozygotic	4–24	Borderline	
			2 F	Monozygotic		Mixed	
	Mixed	2		Dizygotic	6–11	Mixed	50.0
			1 F	Dizygotic	6–11	Mixed	
			1 mixed	Dizygotic			
Lennox, 1947b	Mixed	24		Monozygotic		Seizure discharge	29.0
						Abnormal	58.0
	Mixed with organic seizure etiology	19		Monozygotic		Seizure discharge	0.0
						Abnormality	19.0
	Mixed	23		Dizygotic		Abnormality	17.0
Lennox, 1951	Mixed	61		Monozygotic		Abnormal	61.0
		40		Dizygotic		Abnormal	7.0
	Spike-and-wave	30		Monozygotic		Spike-and-wave	74.0
		11		Dizygotic		Spike-and-wave	27.0
	High voltage slow or spike	8		Monozygotic		High voltage slow or spike	37.0
		14		Dizygotic			0.0
	Slow spike-and-wave	8		Monozygotic		Slow spike-and-wave	25.0
		5		Dizygotic			0.0
Suzuki, 1960	Mixed	72		Monozygotic		Abnormal	73.0
		7		Dizygotic		Abnormal	0.0
Vercelletto and Courjon, 1969	Mixed with both seizure	10		Monozygotic		Epileptiform	60.0

the studies the seizure rate was considerably higher in the monozygotic co-twin than in the dizygotic co-twin.

Clinical Studies

Most of the clinical studies have included multiple seizure types (Lennox, 1974b; Lafon et al., 1956; Braconi, 1962; Vercelletto and Courjon, 1967; Badalyan et al., 1970) and generally have demonstrated a high seizure prevalence in the monozygotic co-twin. In a report of 122 twin pairs of which one twin of each pair was an epileptic proband without a known etiology (Lennox, 1951), 84% of the monozygotic co-twins, but only 10% of the dizygotic co-twins, had seizures. In epileptic probands with a known etiology, 17% of the monozygotic co-twins, but only 8% of the dizygotic co-twins, had suffered seizures.

Similar results were obtained by other investigators (Inouye, 1969; Braconi, 1962; Vercelletto and Courjon, 1967; Badalyan et al., 1970), who found that over half of the monozygotic co-twins had a seizure history, whereas the dizygotic co-twins had a considerably lower rate (Rosenoff et al., 1934; Inouye, 1960; Braconi, 1962; Badalyan et al., 1970).

A review by Koch in 1965 of the twin literature (which included some of the twin studies just mentioned) revealed that 60.8% of 233 monozygotic co-twins, but only 12.3% of 470 dizygotic co-twins, had seizures. When idiopathic seizures were analyzed separately, the seizure rates were similar to those found by Lennox. Although Braconi demonstrated a concordance of 91% for monozygotic twins and 50% for dizygotic twins, this smaller contrast may be due to the small sample. In the larger series that were collected by Gedda and Taterelli (1971) and Conrad (1935) the contrast was considerably greater, with a concordance of 97% and 86% for monozygotic twins in the two series, respectively, and a concordance of 15% and 4% for the dizygotic twins. The rates of acquired epilepsy were considerably lower in both the monozygotic and dizygotic twins when compared with the rates of idiopathic epilepsy, but again the monozygotic twins had a significantly higher concordance. Thus, several of the apparently secondary or organic seizures may have a significant genetic etiology.

The concordance between twins for specific seizure types has also been demonstrated by several investigators. In one of the larger studies, 13 of 26 monozygotic twin pairs, but none of 14 dizygotic pairs, had a concordance for a specific seizure type. (Inouye, 1960). Similar trends were found in the large studies of Conrad (1936a, 1936b), Gedda and Taterelli (1971), and Badalyan et al. (1971), whose complicated study examined many variables, including the neurological and psychiatric status, birth history, and clinical features of the seizures.

The occurrence of different types of seizure has been correlated in twins, including generalized tonic-clonic seizures and absence attacks (Gedda and Taterelli, 1971), photic-induced seizures (Daly and Bickford, 1951), and complex partial seizures (Barslund and Danielsen, 1963). Febrile convulsions have also been studied in two large twin studies, with somewhat conflicting results. Lennox-Buchthal (1971) found that in monozygotic twins with similar neurological development the concordance for febrile convulsions was 80% and the concordance for seizures was generally 100%, whereas Schiottz-Christensen (1972) found only 31% concordance for febrile convulsions between the monozygotic twins and 11% between the dizygotic ones.

To conclude, the twin studies suggest a strong genetic influence on the occurrence of generalized and idiopathic seizures and a lesser genetic influence on symptomatic seizures. The wide differences in seizure rates between monozygotic and dizygotic twins suggest a polygenetic inheritance (Andermann, 1972).

Electroencephalographic Studies

Electroencephalograms of twins have been studied to determine a genetic trend in the tracings (Table 16). The largest series is still the one by Lennox (1947, 1951), who analyzed the electroencephalograms of 61 pairs of twins. At least one twin in each pair studied had epilepsy. Of the monozygotic twins whose seizures had an unknown etiology, epileptiform discharges were present in 33% of their co-twins and other abnormalities were present in 50%. The rates of the dizygotic twins were lower, with 22% having epileptiform discharges and 37% having other abnormalities. However, the significance of these figures is not known because of the high percentage of abnormal electroencephalograms found in dizygotic twins and the somewhat nonspecific abnormalities included in the studies. The epileptiform discharges were not described, but several of the alleged epileptiform discharges might not be significant for epilepsy.

In more recent, although smaller, studies (Inouye, 1960; Suzuki, 1960) a more significant difference was found between the electroencephalograms of monozygotic and dizygotic twins. Approximately 75% of the monozygotic patients demonstrated epileptiform activity, an abnormal tracing, or a history of epilepsy, but less than 10% of the dizygotic twins had these abnormalities (Table 16). The electroencephalogram data, then, is similar to the clinical data and suggests a polygenetic inheritance. A concordance of specific electroencephalogram abnormalities has not been established in large-scale studies of monozygotic and dizygotic twins, but the spike-and-wave pattern at least has been found to have higher concordance in identical twins (Dharmapal and Ramamurthi, 1973).

D. PEDIGREE STUDIES

Several investigators have reported increased seizure rates in specific families (Table 17). Most of the inheritance patterns have been postulated to account for the transmission of the seizure tendency, including a polygenetic model (Tsuboi, 1976), autosomal dominance (Davenport and Weeks, 1911; Hurst, 1963; Andermann, 1972; Meyer, 1973), autosomal dominance with reduced penetrance (Hurst, 1963; Andermann, 1972; Brimani, 1976), and autosomal recessive (Hurst, 1963). Other investigators have described an increased seizure rate in specific families without mentioning a particular inheritance pattern (Koch, 1955; Cordier, 1958; Bancaud, 1969; Beaumanoir et al., 1969; Loiseau and Beaussart, 1969; Catalano, 1973).

TABLE 17. Pedigree studies

Investigator	Epilepsy type	No. of pedigrees	Generations/ pedigree	Family members/ pedigree	Inheritance pattern
Bancaud, 1969	Mixed	1	4	25	?
Beaumanoir et al., 1969	Mixed	3	3–5	7–19	?
Davenport and Weeks, 1911	Mixed	28	4–7	22–142	?
Flood and Collins, 1913	Mixed	6	3–5	24–69	?
Hurst, 1963	Mixed	13	2–3	2–16	Recessive, irregular Dominant, autosomal Dominant
Koch, 1955	Mixed	27	4–8	27–155	?
Meyer, 1973	Febrile convulsions, generalized tonic-clonic	2	3	8–9	Dominant
Wasterlain and Dhaene, 1969	Focal epilepsy	1	4		Recessive

Several specific seizure types have also been identified within a single pedigree. In another review (Newmark and Penry, 1979) photic-induced seizures, pattern seizures, and reading epilepsy are all described as following a familial pattern. Additionally, familial somatosensory partial epilepsy has been found (Wasterlain and Dhaene, 1969) and also familial paroxysmal choreoathetosis (by several investigators). Febrile seizures have been described in three successive generations of two families (Meyer, 1973).

The seizure risk for a family member may increase if more than one other member is involved. Kimball and Hersh (1954) found that the risk of epilepsy in a person who has one sibling with seizures is 9.5%, but if a parent is also involved, the risk becomes 13.5%. In inbred populations the increased familial seizure risk appears to be secondary to a polygenetic inheritance (Utin, 1975a, 1975b). Although the patients within the entire population exhibited different seizure types, the seizure type and age of onset were similar within a single family.

The pedigree studies, although they are suggestive of a genetic influence on seizure occurrence, have not demonstrated a specific inheritance pattern. Andermann (1972) suggested a multifactorial inheritance, based on her studies of electroencephalograms of the relatives of patients with partial seizures, but the results were not sufficiently specific because of the large number of abnormalities in the control population he examined. Rodin et al. (1969) have mentioned that several parameters, including the age of the relative, may be important in the appearance of genetic abnormalities, and Metrakos and Metrakos (1960) have stressed this fact. Also, electroencephalograms, even if they are performed conscientiously and frequently, may not demonstrate abnormal genetic traits.

IV.

Other Factors in the Genetics of Epilepsy

A. AGE

Earlier in this review we discussed the association of epilepsy with certain age groups. Several types of seizure (absence, photosensitive, and febrile) have a specific age-dependent rate of occurrence, and many electroencephalographic abnormalities have age-dependent peaks. Furthermore, as we have said, the proband's age when the seizure disorder begins may be important. In a large group of patients the relatives of probands whose seizures had begun before the age of 5 had almost double the seizure rate of relatives of probands whose seizures had begun between the ages of 5 and 19, and the relatives had almost four times the incidence when proband seizures had begun after the age of 20 (Lennox, 1947). Similar investigations on smaller series of patients did not show a significant correlation between proband age and the age of seizure occurrence in relatives (Soulayrol et al., 1969; Pedersen and Krogh, 1971). However, another small study that restricted the probands to those having tonic-clonic seizures without a known etiology showed that the seizure rate in close relatives of patients whose seizures had begun before the age of 4 was twice that of the relatives of patients whose seizures had begun after the age of 16 (Eisner et al., 1959). A study on focal seizures showed the highest familial seizure rate to be in relatives of probands whose age of onset was 3 to 5, with much lower rates cited for older probands (Andermann, 1972).

This pattern of increased familial seizures when the probands are younger may not be specific for familial seizures. Three factors may be important:

1. Families of patients who develop seizures early are more aware of epileptic manifestations and many recognize subtle signs in other family members.

2. Patients with a late onset of seizures do not always have an accurate history available of the other family members.

3. Patients with a late onset of seizures may have a greater tendency toward symptomatic seizures, which have a lower familial seizure rate.

Some of these factors seem to have influenced the results of a control study by Eisner et al. (1959). A slightly higher seizure rate was found in the relatives of probands under the age of 3 (2.17%) than in the relatives over the age of 16 (1.56%), with intermediate ages having intermediate rates. Although it has been established that some types of seizure have an age-related component, its significance to the genetics of epilepsy as a whole has not been determined.

B. SEX

We have said that studies on the influence of sex factors on the genetics of epilepsy have yielded somewhat mixed results. These analyses have included mixed seizure types (Harvald, 1954; Pedersen and Krogh, 1971; Annegers et al., 1976; Tsuboi and Endo, 1977), generalized tonic-clonic seizures (Tsuboi and Endo, 1977), focal seizures (Andermann, 1972), febrile convulsions (Annegers et al., 1976), and minor motor seizures (Tsuboi and Christian, 1972).

Although several studies did not indicate that the sex of the proband had a significant effect on the familial seizure rate (Harvald, 1954; Pedersen and Krogh, 1971; Andermann, 1972), most of the studies did demonstrate an increased prevalence of seizures in the relatives of female probands (Tsuboi and Christian, 1971; Annegers et al., 1976; Tsuboi and Endo, 1977), particularly the studies of offspring (Tsuboi and Christian, 1971; Annegers et al., 1976) in which factors associated with pregnancy may be important. Electroencephalographic studies analyzing the genetics of centencephalic patterns (Lipinski, 1975) showed no significant difference between male and female probands when seizure rates of offspring were measured.

Several other studies have investigated the sexes of affected relatives having mixed seizures (Harvald, 1951; Ounstead, 1953; Metrakos and Metrakos, 1960; Tsuboi and Endo, 1977), myoclonic or astatic seizures (Doose et al., 1970; Tsuboi and Christian, 1972), and focal seizures (Gerken et al., 1977; Andermann, 1972). Electroencephalographic studies have also been done (Lennox et al., 1940; Andermann, 1972). The results are ambigous. Several investigators found no significant difference between the sexes (Doose et al., 1970; Ounstead, 1953; Andermann, 1972; Gerken et al., 1977; Tsuboi and Endo, 1977), whereas others concluded seizure rates were slightly increased in female relatives (Harvald, 1951; Metrakos and Metrakos, 1960; Kishimoto et al., 1961; Andermann, 1972; Tsuboi and Christian, 1972). This increase is primarily present in studies of probands who have centrencephalic electroencephalographic abnormalities, which are more common in female relatives of female probands (Andermann, 1972). However, the female preponderance toward seizures may be nonspecific since these abnormalities were more common in females of the control population also (Metrakos and Metrakos, 1960). Definite conclusions cannot be reached from other studies because of a lack of controls, (Harvald, 1951; Tsuboi and Christian, 1973).

Knowledge of the influence sex has on the inheritance of epilepsy is somewhat incomplete and the matter may be complicated by other factors. However, in at least some studies a female preponderance of abnormalities is suggested, particularly in certain generalized electroencephalographic disorders that were discussed above (the centrencephalic electroencephalographic pattern and photosensitivity). That female sex hormones may be an added stress factor allowing the expression of a genetic trait is an interesting hypothesis, but has not been proved.

C. SEIZURE CONCORDANCE IN FAMILIAL SEIZURES

The concordance of seizure types has not been extensively investigated except for twin studies. Utin (1975b) noted a similarity of seizure type within individual families, but controls were not examined and specific seizure types were not mentioned. Metrakos and Metrakos (1960) examined patients with centrencephalic tracings and found similar abnormalities in almost 50% of the close relatives within the high-risk age group, 4–16 years. Bray and Wiser (1964) found the midtemporal spike pattern in 36% of the siblings and offspring of probands who had midtemporal spikes, a rate significantly higher than that reported by Heijbel et al. (1975). From the limited electroencephalic studies that have been performed, it can be said that the midtemporal spike and the generalized spike-and-wave are frequently present in affected relatives. Since both abnormalities are strongly associated with the specific seizure types partial seizures and absence attacks, respectively, these seizures may also be present in the affected relatives. However, studies documenting the seizure type rather than the electroencephalographic pattern have not been done in these cases.

Studies that have described one type of seizure have revealed a concordance in close relatives of patients with febrile convulsions (Herlitz et al., 1941; Ounsted et al., 1966; Frantzen et al., 1970; Lennox-Buchthal, 1971; Schiottz-Christensen, 1972). Other seizure types have not been investigated so extensively.

D. SIGNIFICANCE OF FAMILY HISTORY OF EPILEPSY FOR PROGNOSIS

The prognosis of familial epilepsy has not been well established. When a patient has progressive neurological disorders in addition to epilepsy, the prognosis is quite poor, but the prognosis follows that of the basic disorder and not that of the epilepsy. Livingston and Kafar (1947) and Livingston et al. (1947) found that in children who had febrile seizures a family history of epilepsy increased the probability of further seizures, whereas a family history of febrile seizures did not increase future risk. Because of these results, they believe that febrile convulsions and epilepsy are different disorders with a different genetic basis, but that children with an epilepsy trait might initially present with a febrile convulsion. In a recent report from the NINCDS collaborative Perinatal Project (Nelson and Ellenberg, 1978) a similar trend was found, although the increased afebrile seizure risk of children whose family history included epilepsy (7.3%) was considerably lower than that found by Livingston.

  In addition to a family history of epilepsy, the presence of electroencephalographic abnormalities in relatives may be important for the prognosis of febrile convulsions. Nevsimalova et al. (1975) found that electro-encephalographic abnormalities are more frequent in the families of probands who later develop afebrile convulsions. Nevsimalova et al. believe in fact that electroencephalograms should be obtained from the relatives of febrile seizure probands to help determine the prognosis.

  Pedersen and Krogh (1971) analyzed the prognosis of afebrile seizure patients and found that in patients with equivalent phenytoin blood levels, those with positive family histories had poorer control regardless of whether their seizures had a known or an unknown etiology. Although the poorer control may have been secondary to other hereditary disorders, no specific diseases were mentioned. In spite of the fact that this study considered the prognosis in terms of seizure control, correlations between phenytoin blood levels in patients and significant neurological deficits, psychological disorders, or specific seizure types were not performed.

V.

Mechanisms

How the epilepsy trait is transmitted is not yet known, although several mechanisms are possible (McKhann and Shooter, 1969). A number of metabolic and hereditary neurological diseases have been associated with epilepsy, but the large variety of these diseases immensely increases the difficulties of finding a single mechanism responsible for them.

A variety of other pathological and immunological abnormalities have also been examined in familial epileptic patients. Popova et al. (1975) reported antibrain antibodies and brain autoantigens in epileptic patients but did not correlate them with the patients' genetic history. Megrabyan and Amadyan (1976) reported higher than normal LDH isoenzymes in the blood, but the relation of this finding to hereditary seizures remains unclear. The use of histocompatibility antigens may be helpful for identifying individuals at risk for epilepsy. Smeraldi et al. (1975) reported a significant increase of HLA-7 in patients having Lennox-Gastaut syndrome, but other conditions have not been investigated. A specific mechanism for the inheritance of epilepsy as such may never be obtained because of the many causes of epilepsy and its association with a wide variety of clinical disorders. Future investigations, encompassing chromosomal investigations (Walker, 1969), and metabolic and neuroendocrine evaluations that include studies on GABA and neurotransmitters, may add more information, but a direct answer is not presently foreseeable.

VI.

Summary

Evidence of a genetic factor in epilepsy has been obtained from several sources. Indirect evidence includes (1) the presence of nonspecific familial electroencephalographic patterns, (2) genetic seizures in many species, and (3) hereditary diseases in which epilepsy is a symptom. More direct evidence has been obtained from clinical examinations of epileptic probands and their relatives. If individuals who have suffered a single seizure are included, 30 to 40% of unselected seizure patients will have a positive family history and up to 10% of their offspring may have epilepsy, with the highest rate present in the offspring of affected mothers. A lower but still significant rate appears in the siblings and parents of probands, but accurate accounts are more difficult to obtain with these two groups than with offspring.

When patients manifest generalized seizure disorders, generalized tonic-clonic seizures, absence attacks, photosensitive epilepsy, and febrile convulsions, the rate of seizures in their relatives is even higher, often twice the rate found in the relatives of unselected patients. In patients who have partial and symptomatic seizures, a genetic trend has not been definitely shown.

The electroencephalographic data are supportive of a theory that genetic factors play an important role in epilepsy. Specific patterns frequently associated with epilepsy, including generalized spike-and-wave discharges, the centrotemporal spike, and the photoconvulsive response, appear at high rates in susceptible relatives. Such findings must be qualified, however, because of their presence in controls, and further evaluation is required to determine the clinical significance of these electroencephalographic patterns. Whether these abnormalities represent a subclinical seizure trait is currently not known.

Twin studies not only corroborate theories of a genetic factor in epilepsy; they also suggest an inheritance pattern. The high rate of seizures found in monozygotic twins (up to 90%) contrasted with the much lower rate in dizygotic twins (10–15%) implies a polygenetic inheritance. Because environmental factors may contribute to the disparity between monozygotic and dizygotic twins, this pattern of inheritance has not been proved.

Areas still requiring evaluation are: (1) the importance of a family history of epilepsy in establishing a proband's seizure control, (2) the mechanisms of transmission of the genetic trait, and (3) the significance of electroencephalographic abnormalities in relatives.

References

Aicardi J, Bancaud J, Beaussart M, Cohadon F, Courjon J, Favel P, Gastaut H, Kerfriden R, Lectercq E, Lerique A, Loiseau P, Miribel J, Passouant P, Roger J, Rohmer F, Sallou C, Schneider J, Soulayrol R, Thieffrey S, and Vercelletto P. General conclusions concerning familial factors in epilepsy. *Epilepsia* 10:65–68, 1969.

Alstrom CH. A study of epilepsy in its clinical, social and genetic aspects. *Acta Psychiatr Kbh* 63:284, 1950.

Alvarez WC. Percentage breakdown for inheritance of epilepsy, in Alvarez WC (ed): *Nerves in Collision.* New York: Pyramid House, 1972, pp 121–132.

Andermann ED. Focal epilepsy and related disorders: genetic, metabolic, and prognostic studies. *Ph.D. Thesis,* McGill University, 1972.

Andermann E, and Metrakos JD. EEG studies of relatives of probands with focal epilepsy who have been treated surgically. *Epilepsia* 10:415–420, 1969.

Andermann E, Remillard GM, Goyer C, Blitzer L, Andermann F, and Barbeau A. Genetic and family studies on Friedreich's ataxia. *Can J Neurol Sci* 3:287–301, 1976.

Annegers JF, Hauser WA, Elveback LR, Anderson VE, and Kurland LT. Seizure disorders in offspring of parents with a history of seizures—a maternal-paternal difference. *Epilepsia* 17:1–9, 1976.

Aschner B, Heves HP, and Tschabitscher H. The inheritance of progressive muscular dystrophy and disposition to convulsions. *Nervenarzt* 35:501–504, 1964.

Atkeson FW, Ibsen HC, and Eldridge F. Inheritance of an epileptic type character in Brown Swiss cattle. *J Hered* 35:45–48, 1944.

Badalyan LD, Gorlina IS, Leibovich FA, Oradovskaya IV, and Yakovleva LF. Clinical, genetic, and electroencephalographic study of epilepsy in twins. *Zh Nevropatol Psikhiatr* 70:329–336, 1970.

Bancaud J. Familial epilepsy through four generations. *Epilepsia* 10:77–82, 1969.

Barolin GS, and Pateisky K. Siblings with Unverricht Lundborg myo-

REFERENCES

clonic epilepsy: A familial and longitudinal investigation. *Electro-encephalogr Clin Neurophysiol* 27:211–212, 1969.

Barr HS, and Galindo J. The Borjeson-Forssman-Lehmann syndrome. *J Ment Defic Res* 9:125–130, 1965.

Barslund I, and Danielson J. Temporal epilepsy in monozygotic twins. *Epilepsia* 4:138–150, 1963.

Beaumanoir A, Martin F, and Souza D. Genetic generalized epilepsy. A follow-up study of 4 patients born between 1880 and 1892. *Epilepsia* 10:69–75, 1969.

Beaussart M. Epilepsy and heredity. *Rev Neuropsychiatr Infant* 19:341–350, 1971.

Beaussart M, and Loiseau P. Hereditary factors in a random population of 5,200 epileptics. *Epilepsia* 10:55–63, 1969.

Benezech M, and Noel B. 47 XYY genotype and neurology. *Bordeaux Med* 8:961–988, 1975.

Benezech M, Noel B, Messager A, Lazarini H-J, and Doignon J. Agressivite, debilite mentale et epilepsie chez un sujet de caryotype 47 XXY/48 XXY. *Rev Neuropsychiatr Infant* 20:773–775, 1972.

Beteta E. Paroxysmal activity in 2,000 EEGs in Peru. *Clin EEG* 3:145–148, 1972.

Bielefelt SW, Redman HC, and McClellan RO. Sire and sex related differences in rates of epileptiform seizures in a purebred Beagle dog colony. *Am J Vet Res* 32:2039–2048, 1971.

Bignami A, Maccagnani F, Zappella M, and Tingey AH. Familial infantile spasms and hypsarrhythmia associated with leucodystrophy. *J Neurol Psychiatr* 29:129–134, 1966.

Bjerre I, and Corelius E. Benign familial neonatal convulsions. *Acta Paediatr Scand* 57:557–561, 1968.

Blom S, Heijbel J, and Bergfars PG. Benign epilepsy of children with centrotemporal electroencephalographic foci. Prevalence and follow-up study of forty patients. *Epilepsia* 13:609–619, 1972.

Boggan WO, and Seiden LS. Dopa reversal of reserpine enhancement of audiogenic seizure susceptibility in mice. *Physiol Behav* 6:215–217, 1971.

Book JA. A genetic and neuropsychiatric investigation of a North-Swedish population with special regard to schizophrenia and mental deficiency. II. Mental deficiency and convulsive disorders. *Acta Genet* 4:345–408, 1953.

REFERENCES

Borjeson M, Forssman H, and Lehmann O. An X-linked, recessively inherited syndrome characterized by grave mental deficiency, epilepsy, and endocrine disorder. *Acta Med Scand* 171:13–21, 1962.

Braconi L. Twin research in epilepsy. *Acta Genet* 11:138–157, 1962.

Brady RO. Inherited metabolic diseases of the nervous system. *Science* 193:733–739, 1976.

Bray PF. Temporal lobe syndrome in children. A longitudinal review. *Pediatrics* 29:617–628, 1962.

Bray PF, and Wiser WC. Evidence for a genetic etiology of temporal-central abnormalities in focal epilepsy. *N. Engl J Med* 271:926–933, 1964.

Bray PF, and Wiser WC. Hereditary characteristics of familial temporal-central focal epilepsy. *Pediatrics* 36:207–211, 1965a.

Bray PF, and Wiser WC. The relation of focal to diffuse epileptiform EEG discharges in genetic epilepsy. *Arch Neurol* 13:222–238, 1965b.

Bridge EM. *Epilepsy and Convulsive Disorders In Children,* New York: McGraw-Hill, 1949.

Brimani D. A propos de l'heredite epileptique chez certains enfants comitiaux. *Encephale* 2:177–186, 1976.

Browne TR, Penry JK, Porter RJ, and Dreifuss FE. Responsiveness before, during, and after spike-wave paroxysms. *Neurology* 24:659–665, 1974.

Buscaino GA, Guazzi GC, and Barbieri FA et al. Ultrastructural and histochemical studies on the Unverricht Lundborg syndrome. Description of a family from the south of Italy. *Acta Neurol* 28:291–322, 1973.

Catalano F. Remarks on the pathogenesis of so-called idiopathic epilepsy. *Acta Neurol* 28:183–207, 1973.

Chiofalo N, Fuentes A, and Muranda M. Progressive myoclonus epilepsy associated with a disorder of iron metabolism. *Neurochirugia* 32:71–77, 1974.

Cobb S. Special article. Causes of epilepsy. *Arch Neurol Psychiatr* 27:1245–1263, 1932.

Collins RL, and Fuller JL. Audiogenic seizure prone (asp): A gene affection behavior in linkage group VIII of the mouse. *Science* 162:1137–1139, 1968.

Conrad K. Erbanlage und epilepsie. Untersuchungen an einer serie von 253 zwillingspaaren. *Z Neurol Psychiatr* 153:271–326, 1935.

REFERENCES

Conrad K. Erbanlage und epilepsie. II. Ein beitrag zur zwillingskasuistik: die Konkordanten eineiigen. *Z Gesamte Neurol Psychiatr* 155:254–297, 1936a.

Conrad K. Erbanlage und epilepsie. III. Ein beitrag zur zwillingskasuistik: die diskordanten eineiigen. *Z Gesamte Neurol Psychiatr* 155:509–542, 1936b.

Conrad K. Erbanlage und epilepsie. IV. Ergebnisse einer nachkommenschaftsuntersuchung an epileptikern. *Z Gesamte Neurol Psychiatr* 159:521–581, 1937.

Cordier J. "Genetic" epilepsy. *Acta Neurol Belg* 58:10–25, 1958.

Cox B, and Lomax P. Brain amines and spontaneous epileptic seizures in the mongolian gerbil. *Pharmacol Biochem Behav* 4:263–267, 1976.

Crawford RD. Epileptiform seizures in domestic fowl. *J Hered* 61:188, 1970.

Currie S, Heathfield KWG, Henson RA, and Scott DF. Clinical course and prognosis of temporal lobe epilepsy. A survey of 666 patients. *Brain* 94:173–190, 1971.

Daly D, and Bickford RG. Electroencephalographic studies of identical twins with photo-epilepsy. *Electroencephalogr Clin Neurophysiol* 3:245–249, 1951.

Davenport CB, and Weeks DF. A first study of inheritance of epilepsy. *J Nerv Ment Dis* 38:641–670, 1911.

Degen R. Probleme der atiologie und elektroenzephalographie der kindlichen epilepsie. *Dtsch Ges.wesen* 27:71–76, 1972.

Degen R. Die wertigkeit der genetik und exogener faktoren in der entstehung kindlicher epilepsien. *Munch Med Wochenschr* 117:465–472, 1975.

Degen R, Arnold H, and Bruhn B. The genetics of infantile spasms. A clinical and electroencephalographic study of families. *Schw Arch Neurol Neurochir Psychiatr* 110:189–203, 1972.

Delaveleye R. The problem of heredity in epilepsy. *Rev Neuropsychiatr Infant* 13:379–399, 1965.

Dharmapal N, and Ramamurthi B. Epilepsy in twins. *Proc Inst Neurol* 3:97–102, 1973.

Dice LR. Inheritance of waltzing and of epilepsy in mice of the genus *Peromyscus*. *J Mammal* 16:25–35, 1935.

Diebold K. Four genetic and clinical types of progressive myoclonus epilepsies. *Arch Psychiatr Nervenkr* 215:362–375, 1972.

REFERENCES

Diebold K, Kastner M, and Penin H. Progressive myoclonus epilepsy in two siblings and 5 cases with dyssynergia cerebellaris myoclonica in several generations of a kinship, a clinical and genetic study. *Nervenarzt* 45:595–601, 1974.

Dobson R, and Ohnuki Y. Chromosomal abnormalities in a child with a convulsive disorder. *Lancet* 2:627–630, 1961.

Doose H. On the genetics of myoclonic-astatic petit mal. *Electroencephalogr Clin Neurophysiol* 31:410, 1971.

Doose H, Eckel U, and Volzke E. Convulsions after smallpox vaccination. *Z Kinderheilk* 103:214–236, 1968.

Doose H, and Gerken H. On the genetics of EEG-anomalies in childhood. IV. Photoconvulsive reaction. *Neuropaeditrie* 4:162–171, 1973.

Doose H, and Gerken H. The genetics of EEG anomalies. *Handbook of Electroencephalogr Clin Neurophysiol* 15:14–18, 1972a.

Doose H, and Gerken H. Possibilities and limitations of epilepsy prevention in siblings of epileptic children, in Parsonage MJ (ed): *Prevention of Epilepsy and Its Consequences,* Proceedings of the Fifth European Symposium on Epilepsy, London, England: July 17–19, 1972b, pp 32–35.

Doose H, Gerken H, Kiefer R, and Volzke E. Genetic factors in childhood epilepsy with focal sharp waves. II. EEG findings in patients and siblings. *Neuropaediatrie* 8:10–20, 1977.

Doose H, Gerken H, Leonhardt R, Volzke E, and Volz C. Centrencephalic myoclonic-astatic petit mal. Clinical and genetic investigations *Neuropaediatrie* 2:59–78, 1970.

Doose H, Gerken H, and Volzke E. Elektrencephalographische untersuchungen uber die genetik zentrencephaler epilepsien. *Z Kinderheilk* 101:242–257, 1967.

Doose H, Gerken H, and Volzke E. On the genetics of EEG-anomalies in childhood. I. Abnormal theta rhythms. *Neuropaediatrie* 3:386–401, 1972.

Dumon-Radermecker M. Very late forms of amaurotic idiocy in a kindred with congenital oligophrenia with epilepsy. *Acta Neurol Belg* 65:779–807, 1965.

Duffner PK, and Cohen ME. Infantile spasms associated with histidinemia. *Neurology* 25:195–197, 1975.

Dustman RE, and Beck EC. The visually evoked potentials in twins. *Electroencephalogr Clin Neurophysiol* 19:570–575, 1965.

REFERENCES

Echeverria MG. Marriage and hereditariness of epileptics. *Am J Insanity* 37:177–216, 1880.

Eisner V, Pauli LL, and Livingston S. Hereditary aspects of epilepsy. *Bull Johns Hopkins Hosp* 105:245–271, 1959.

Eisner V, Pauli LL, and Livingston S. Epilepsy in the families of epileptics. *J Pediatr* 56:347–354, 1960.

Evans JH. Post-traumatic epilepsy. *Neurology* (Minneap) 12:665–674, 1962.

Falco MJ, Barker J, and Wallace ME. The genetics of epilepsy in the British Alsatian. *J Small Anim Pract* 15:685–692, 1974.

Falconer MA. Genetic and retarded aetiological factors in temporal lobe epilepsy. A review. *Epilepsia* 12:13–31, 1971.

Flood E, and Collins M. A study of heredity in epilepsy. *Am J Insanity* 69:585–603, 1913.

Forssman H, and Akesson HO. Extra Y chromosomes and epilepsy. *Humangenetik* 7:251–252, 1969.

Frantzen E, Lennox-Buchthal M, and Nygaard A. Febrile convulsions—a follow-up and genetic study. *Excerpta Medica* (Amsterdam) 193:57, 1969.

Frantzen E, Lennox-Buchthal M, Nygaard A, and Stene J. A genetic study of febrile convulsions. *Neurology* 20:909–917, 1970.

Frezza M, Vettore L, Perona G, and DeSandre G. Familial encephalopathy associated with a small metacentric chromosome. *Folia Hered Pathol (Milano)* 15:107–113, 1966.

Gaches J, Koupernik C, Poissonnier M, and Sallou C. Epilepsy and heredity: A working hypothesis. *Concours Med* 89:6243–6251, 1967.

Gastaut H. On genetic transmission of epilepsies. *Epilepsia* 10:3–6, 1969.

Gastaut H, Papy JJ, Toga M, Murisasco A, and Dubois, X. Epilepsy in renal insufficiency and accidental epileptic seizures during hemodialysis (artificial kidney). *Rev Electroencephalogr Neurophysiol Clin* 1:151–162, 1971.

Gastaut H, Tassinari CA, Roger J, Soulayrol R, Saint Jean M, Regis H, Bernard R, Pinsard N, and Dravet C. Juvenile epileptic encephalopathy associated with diffuse slow spike wave activity ("atypical petit mal"; Lennox syndrome). *Rec Prog Med (Roma)* 45:117–146, 1968.

Gayral L, and Gayral J. Epilepsy and hereditary spinocerebellar degeneration. *J Genet Hum* 17:127–136, 1969.

Gedda L, and Tatarelli R. Essential isochronic epilepsy in MZ twin pairs. *Acta Genet Med* 20:380–383, 1971.

Gerken H, and Doose H. On the genetics of EEG anomalies in childhood. II. Occipital 2–4/s rhythms. *Neuropaediatrie* 3:437–454, 1972.

Gerken H, Kiefer R, Doose H, and Volzke E. Genetic factors in childhood epilepsy with focal sharp waves. I. Clinical data and familial morbidity for seizures. *Neuropaediatrie* 8:3–9, 1977.

Giove C. Alcoholic epilepsy. *Osped Psichiat* 32:195–266, 1965.

Gowers WR. *Epilepsy and Other Chronic Convulsive Diseases*, New York: William Wood, 1881.

Graveleau D. Febrile convulsions. *Concours Med* 96:5773–5785, 1974.

Green JB. Epilepsy in inherited mental and motor disorders. *Psychiatr Forum* 4:39–45, 1973.

Gross-Selbeck G, and Doose H. Essential myoclonus in childhood (paramyoclonus multiplex). *Neuropaediatrie* 6:117–125, 1975.

Guazzi GC, Ghetti B, Barbieri F, and Cecio A. Myoclonus epilepsy with cherry red spot in adult: A peculiar form of mucopolysaccharidosis. A clinical, genetical, chemical, and ultrastructural study. *Acta Neurol* 28:542–548, 1973.

Hall C. Genetic differences in fatal audiogenic seizures between two inbred strains of house mice. *J Hered* 38:3–6, 1947.

Hamaguchi K, Sugiyama Y, and Sakae F. Kinesthetic reflex epilepsy. *Clin Neurol* (Tokyo) 9:281–290, 1969.

Harvald B. Hereditary factors in epilepsy. *Med Clin North Am* 58:345–348, 1958.

Harvald B. *Heredity In Epilepsy. An Electroencephalographic Study of Relatives of Epileptics*, Copenhagen: Ejnar Munksgaard, 1954.

Harvald B. On the genetic prognosis of epilepsy. *Acta Psychiatr Neurol* 26:339–357, 1951.

Hegreberg GA, and Padgett GA. Inherited progressive epilepsy of the dog with comparisons to Lafora's disease of man. *Fed Proc* 35:1202–1205, 1976.

Heijbel J, Blom S, and Rasmuson M. Benign epilepsy of childhood with centrotemporal EEG foci: A genetic study. *Epilepsia* 16:285–293, 1975.

Herlitz G. Studient uber die sogennanten initialen fieberkrampfe bei kindern. *Acta Paediatr Scand* 29(Suppl 1), 1941.

Hertz L, Schousboe A, Formby B, and Lennox-Buchthal M. Some

age dependent biochemical changes in mice susceptible to seizures. *Epilepsia* 15:619–631, 1974.

Hirayama K. Metabolism of acid soluble nucleotides and other phosphorus compounds in the brain with special reference to convulsive activity. *Psychiatr Neurol Jap* 65:842–855, 1963.

Hirooka M, Ohno T, and Kubota N. Hereditary hematuria associated with mental retardation, convulsions, abnormal EEG and ocular abnormalities. *Tokohu J Exp Med* 98:199–211, 1969.

Hoeppner T, Morrell F, and Hoeppner JA. Skin scarring and posttraumatic epilepsy. *Neurology* (Minneap) 23:437, 1973.

Hohenboken WD, and Nellhaus G. Inheritance of audiogenic seizures in the rabbit. *J Hered* 61:107–112, 1970.

Holowach J, Renda YA, and Wapner I. Psychomotor seizures in childhood. A clinical study of 120 cases. *J Pediatr* 59:339–346, 1961.

Holowach J, Thurston DL, and O'Leary J. Jacksonian seizures in infancy and childhood. *J Pediatr* 52:670–686, 1958.

Hommes FA, De Groat CJ, Wilmink CW, and Jonxis JHP: Carbamylphosphate synthetase deficiency in an infant with severe cerebral damage. *Arch Dis Child* 44:688–693, 1969.

Horak F. Some genetic problems of audiogenic epilepsy in rats and rabbits. *Comparative and Cellular Pathophysiology of Epilepsy,* Amsterdam: Exc Med FDN, 1966, pp 325–330.

Houston, AB, Brodie MJ, Moore MR, Thompson GG, and Stephenson JB. Hereditary coproporphyria and epilepsy. *Arch Dis Child* 52:646–650, 1977.

Hrbek A: Febrile convulsions in childhood. *Ann Paediatr Basel* 188:162–182, 1957.

Hudgins RL, and Corbin KB. An uncommon seizure disorder: Familial paroxysmal choreoathetosis. *Brain* 89:199–204, 1966.

Hurst LA. Problems in the genetics of epilepsy. *S Afr Med J* 37:208–211, 1963.

Hurst LA. Genetic aspects of epilepsy. *S Afr Med J* 48:603–605, 1974.

Inouye E. Genetics of epilepsy: A review. *Adv Neurol Sci* 12:414–418, 1968.

Inouye E. Observations on forty twin index cases with chronic epilepsy and their co-twins. *J Nerv Ment Dis* 130:401–416, 1960.

Ioanitiu D, Maximilian C, and Florea I. Genetic aspects of epilepsy in an isolated population with endemic thyropathic dystrophy (endemic goiter). *Rev Roum Endocrinol* 3:73–81, 1966.

Jancar J. Norrie's disease. Recessive, sex linked, progressive, oculocerebral degeneration. *Clin Genet (Kbh)* 1:353–356, 1970.

Janeway R, Ravens JR, Pearce LA, Odor DL, and Suzuki K. Progressive myoclonus epilepsy with Lafora inclusion bodies. I. Clinical, genetic, histopathologic, and biochemical aspects. *Arch Neurol* 16:565–582, 1967.

Jensen I. Genetic factors in temporal lobe epilepsy. *Acta Neurol Scand* 52:381–394, 1975.

Jeras J, and Tividar I. *Epilepsies in Children.* The University Press of New England, Hanover, New Hampshire, 1973.

Kagawa K. A genetic study of febrile convulsions. *Brain Dev* 7:369–384, 1975.

Kallmann FJ, and Sander G. The genetics of epilepsy, in Hoch PH and Knight RP (eds): *Epilepsy. Psychiatric Aspects of Convulsive Disorders,* New York: Hafner Publishing Co., 1947, pp 27–41.

Kimball OP: On the inheritance of epilepsy. *Wis Med J* 53:271–276, 1954.

Kimball OP, and Hersh AH. The genetics of epilepsy. *Acta Genet Med Gemollol (Roma)* 4:131–142, 1955.

Kishimoto K, Kurita A, and Amano S. A hereditary study of the electroencephalography on some endogenous nervous diseases. *Nagoya Med J* 7:61–65, 1961.

Klein D, Mumenthaler M, Kraus-Ruppert R, and Rallo E. A Valais family affected with progressive myoclonic epilepsy and retinitis pigmentosa. A clinical, genetic, and pathologic study. *Rev Neurol* 19:180–181, 1968a.

Klein D, Mumenthaler M, Kraus-Ruppert R, and Rallo E. A large family of Valais affected with progressive myoclonic epilepsy and with retinitis pigmentosa. Clinical, genetic and pathologic study. *Humangenetic* 6:237–252, 1968b.

Koch G. *Proneness To Seizures (Its Genetic Basis),* Roma: Gregorio Mendel, 1955.

Koch G. Genetics of epilepsy. *Med Welt* 25:1389–1396, 1965.

Koch G. The hereditary character of the epilepsies. *Psychiatr Neurol Neurochir* 66:153–183, 1963.

REFERENCES

Kolpakov VG, and Galaktionov OK. A genetic and biochemical study of audiogenic epilepsy. III. A comparative study of the biochemical mechanisms of audiogenic epilepsy in rats of the Krushinskii Molodkin strain and in DBA mice. *Sov Genet* 6:1598–1604, 1973.

Korten JJ, Notermans SLH, Frenken CWGM, Gabreels FJM, and Jooste EM. Familial essential myoclonus. *Brain* 97:131–138, 1974.

Kramer W, and Makkink B. Multiple endocrine adenomas (Lloyd's syndrome) and psychomotor epilepsy. *Neurology (Minneap)* 11:571–577, 1961.

Kruse R. Sleep epilepsy in childhood. Grand mal and focal seizures. *Nervenartz* 35:200–207, 1964.

Kuhlo W, Heintel H, and Vogel F. The 4–5 c/sec rhythm. *Electroencephalogr Clin Neurophysiol* 26:613–618, 1969.

Kunze J, Doose H, and Folksdorf M. Dysplasia epilepsia syndrome in a patient with ring chromosome 21. *Neuropadiatrie* 6:398–402, 1975.

Kurokawa M, Naruse H, and Kato M. Metabolic studies on *ep* mouse, a special strain with convulsive predisposition, in Tokizane T and Schade JP (eds): *Progress in Brain Research Vol 21A, Correlative Neurosciences Part A—Fundamental Mechanisms,* 1966, pp 112–130.

Lacy JR, and Penry JK. *Infantile Spasms.* Raven Press, New York, 1976.

Lafon R, Passouant P, Faure JL, and Minvielle J. Epilepsy in twins. Clinical, electroencephalographic and psychologic study of 7 pairs of homozygous epileptic twins. *Montpellier Med* 49:56–75, 1956.

Lennox MA. Febrile convulsions in childhood. A clinical and electroencephalographic study. *Am J Dis Child* 78:868–882, 1949.

Lennox WG. The multiple causes of seizures in the individual epileptic patient. *N Engl J Med* 209:386–389, 1933.

Lennox WG. The heredity of epilepsy as told by relatives and twins. *JAMA* 146:529–536, 1951.

Lennox WG. The genetics of epilepsy. *Am J Psychiatr* 103:457–462, 1947a.

Lennox WG. Sixty-six twin pairs affected by seizures. *Assoc Rev Nerv Ment Dis Proc* 26:11–34, 1947b.

Lennox WG, and Davis JP. Clinical correlates of the fast and slow spike-waves electroencephalograph. *Pediatrics* 5:626–644, 1950.

Lennox WG, Gibbs EL, and Gibbs FA. The inheritance of epilepsy

REFERENCES

as revealed by the electroencephalograph. *JAMA* 113:1002–1003, 1939.

Lennox WG, Gibbs EL, and Gibbs FA. Inheritance of cerebral dyrhythmia and epilepsy. *Arch Neurol Psychiatr* 44:1155–1183, 1940.

Lennox WG, Gibbs EL, and Gibbs FA. Twins, brain waves and epilepsy. *Arch Neurol Psychiatr* 47:702–706, 1942.

Lennox WG, Gibbs EL, and Gibbs FA. The brain-wave pattern, an hereditary trait. Evidence from 74 "normal" pairs of twins. *J Hered* 36:233–243, 1945.

Lennox-Buchthal M. Febrile and nocturnal convulsions in monozygotic twins. *Epilepsia* 12:147–156, 1971.

Lennox-Buchthal MA. Febrile convulsions. A reappraisal. *Electroencephalogr Clin Neurophysiol* (Suppl 32), 1973.

Lindsay JMM. Genetics and epilepsy: A model from critical path analysis. *Epilepsia* 12:47–54, 1971.

Lipinski C, Benninger C, Janz D, Scheffner D, Seminario P, and Stolzis L. Historical data and EEG findings in children of epileptic and nonepileptic patients, in Janz D (ed): *Epileptology,* Proceedings of the Seventh International Symposium on Epilepsy in Berlin (West), June 1975, Thieme, Berlin, 1975, pp 29–32.

Little SC, and Weaver NK. Epilepsy in twins. An analysis of five twin pairs, with electroencephalographic studies. *Am J Dis Child* 79:223–232, 1950.

Livingston S, Bridge, EM, and Kajdi L. Febrile convulsions: A clinical study with special reference of heredity and prognosis. *J Pediatr* 31:509–512, 1947.

Livingston S, and Kajar L. Important of heredity in the prognosis of febrile convulsions. *Am J Dis Child* 69:324–325, 1945.

Loiseau P, and Beaussart M. Hereditary factors in partial epilepsy. *Epilepsia* 10:23–31, 1969.

Lund M. *Epilepsy In Association With Intractable Tumour. Acta Psychiatr Scand* 1952, 81:149 pp.

Lundin G, Moller A. Views on the question of the sterilization of epileptics. *Acta Psychiatr Scand* 26:177–189, 1951.

Lupu I, Macovei Lupu M, Cocinschi R, and Fratila A. Febrile infantile convulsions. Electroclinical contributions. *Electroencephalogr Clin Neurophysiol* 30:360–361, 1971.

REFERENCES

Lykken DT, Tellegen A, Thorkelson K. Genetic determination of EEG frequency spectra. *Biol Psychol* 1:245–259, 1974.

MacIntosh RR. The significance of fits in eclampsia. *J Obstet Gynaec Brit Emp* 59:197–201, 1952.

Malin JP. Differential diagnosis of hereditary spastic spinal paralysis. *Nervenarzt* 47:661–668, 1976.

Malzberg B. Order of birth and size of family among epileptics. *Acta Psychiatr Scand* 49:341–352, 1973.

Marburg O, and Helfand M. Analysis of one hundred cases of epilepsy. *J Nerv Ment Dis* 104:465–473, 1946.

Matthes A. Genetic studies in epilepsy, in Gastaut H, Jasper H, Bancaud J, and Waltregny A (eds): *The Physiopathogenesis of the Epilepsies,* Springfield: CC Thomas, 1969, pp 26–30.

Matthes A, and Weber H. Clinical and electroencephalographic family studies in pyknolepsies. *Dtsch Med Wochenschr* 93:429–435, 1968.

Mattila R (ed). Proceedings of the 22nd Scandinavian Congress of Neurology, Turku, 1978. Mankssgaard, Copenhagen, 1978.

McKhann GM, and Shooter EM. Genetics of seizure susceptibility, in Jasper AH, Ward AA, and Pope A (eds): *Basic Mechanisms of the Epilepsies,* Boston: Little, Brown and Co., 1969, pp 689–708.

Megrabyan AA, and Amadyan MG. Clinico pathophysiological aspects of hereditary predisposition to epilepsy in children and adolescents. *Zh Nevropat Psikhiat Korsakov* 76:422–426, 1976.

Menkes JH. *Textbook of Child Neurology.* New York: Lea & Febiger, 1974.

Menkes JH, Andrews JM, and Cancilla PA. The cerebroretinal degenerations. *J Pediatr* 79:183–196, 1971.

Metrakos JD. Heredity as an etiological factor in convulsive disorders, in Fields WS and Desmond MM (eds): *Disorders of the Developing Nervous System,* Springfield: CC Thomas, 1961, pp 23–41.

Metrakos JD, and Metrakos K. Genetics of convulsive disorders. I. Introduction, problems, methods, and base lines. *Neurology* 10:228–240, 1960.

Metrakos JD, Metrakos K. Genetic studies in clinical epilepsy, in Jasper HH, Ward AA, and Pope A (eds): *Basic Mechanisms of the Epilepsies.* Boston: Little, Brown and Co., 1969, pp 700–708.

Metrakos JD, and Metrakos K. Genetic factors in epilepsy. *Epilepsy Mod Probl Pharmacopsychiatr* 4:71–86, 1970.

REFERENCES

Metrakos JD, and Metrakos K. Genetic factors in the epilepsies. *NINDS Monograph No. 14,* DHEW Publication No. (NIH) 73–390, Bethesda, 1972, pp 97–102.

Metrakos JD, Metrakos K, Polizos P, and Valle F. Genetics and onto-genesis of the centrencephalic EEG. *Electroencephalogr Clin Neurophysiol* 21:404, 1966.

Metrakos K, and Metrakos JD. Genetics of convulsive disorders. II. Genetics and electroencephalographic studies in centrencephalic epilepsy. *Neurology* 11:414–483, 1961a.

Metrakos K, and Metrakos JD. Is the centrencephalic EEG inherited as a dominant. *Electroencephalogr Clin Neurophysiol* 13:289, 1961b.

Meyer JG. On the inheritance of spike wave complexes and febrile seizures in three generations. *Dtsch Med Wochenschr* 98:1717–1719, 1973.

Meyer JG, Holzinger H, and Urban K. Epileptic seizures in alcoholic predelirium. Clinical and electroencephalographic studies on the differentiation of genetic conditioned attack predisposition and epilepsy. *Nervenarzt* 47:375–379, 1976.

Millichap JG: *Febrile Convulsions.* New York: Macmillan, 1968.

Millichap JG, Bickford RG, Klass DW, and Backus RE. Infantile spasms, hypsarrhythmia and mental retardation. A study of aetiologic factors in 61 patients. *Epilepsia* 3:188–197, 1962.

Millichap JG, Madsen JA, and Alldort LM. Studies in febrile seizures. V. Clinical and electroencephalographic study in unselected patients. *Neurology (Minneap)* 10:643–653, 1960.

Mirimanoff P. Hereditary spongy degeneration of the central nervous system in children (Canavan, van Bogaert et Bertrand). *J Neurol Sci* 28:159–185, 1976.

Mollica F, Mazzone D, and Pavone L. The familial incidence of febrile convulsions. *Clin Pediatr (Phila)* 28:1–8, 1973.

Muller K, Arnold H, Bruhn B et al. Familial predisposition in focal epilepsy. *Schw Arch Neurol Neuropsychiatr* 113:45–55, 1973.

Muskens LJJ. Heredity and other predisposing factors in epilepsy. *Epilepsy.* New York: William Wood Co., 1928, pp 271–273.

Naquet R, and Lanoir J. Essay on antiepileptic drug activity in experimental animals: special tests, in Radouco-Thomas J, and Mercier J (eds): *International Encyclopedia of Pharmacology and Therapeutics/ Anticonvulsant Drugs, Vol I,* 1973, pp 67–122.

Nelson KB, and Ellenberg JH. Prognosis in children with febrile seizures. *Pediatrics* 61:720–727, 1978.

Nevsimalova S, Dittrich J, Roth B, and Rothova N. Febrile convulsions. A clinical, genealogic and electroencephalographic family study. *CS Neurol Neurochir* 38:207–215, 1975.

Newmark ME, and Penry JK. *Photosensitivity and epilepsy: A review.* Raven Press, New York, 1979, 230 pp.

Nielsen J, and Pedersen E. Electro-encephalographic findings in patients with Klinefelter's syndrome and the XXY syndrome. *Acta Neurol Scand* 45:87–94, 1969.

Ortiz de Zarote JC. Heredity in epilepsy. *Rev Assoc Med Argent* 82:308–314, 1968.

Ounsted C. The factor of inheritance in convulsive disorders in childhood. *Proc R Soc Med* 45:37/865–40/868, 1952.

Ounsted C. The sex ratio in convulsive disorders with a note on single-sex sibships. *J. Neurol Neurosurg Psychiatr* 16:267–274, 1953.

Ounsted C, Lindsay J, and Norman R. Biological factors in temporal lobe epilepsy. *Clinics In Development Medicine #22.* London: The Spastics Society Medical Education and Information, in association with William Heinemann Medical Books, Ltd., 1966.

Pampus I, and Seidenfaden I. Posttraumatic epilepsy. *Fortschr Neurol Psychiatr* 42:329–384, 1974.

Paskind HA. Extramural patients with epilepsy. With special references to the frequency absence of deterioration. *Arch Neurol Psychiatr* 28:370–385, 1932.

Paskind HA, and Brown M. Frequency of epilepsy in offspring of persons with epilepsy. With special reference to differences between institutional and extramural patients. *Arch Neurol Psychiatr* 36:1045–1048, 1936.

Paskind HA, and Brown M. Hereditary factors in epilepsy. Differences between deteriorated and nondeteriorated patients. *JAMA* 108:1599–1601, 1937.

Pedersen E. Postencephalic epilepsy. *Epilepsia* 5:43–50, 1964.

Pedersen HE, and Krogh E. The prognostic consequences of familial predisposition and sex in epilepsy. *Acta Neurol Scand* 47:105–116, 1971.

Penfield W, and Paine K. Results of surgical therapy for focal epileptic seizures. *Can Med Assoc J* 73:515–531, 1955.

REFERENCES

Pescia G. Epileptogenous encephalopathy of early onset, with recessive inheritance in two families of an isolated Valais community (with pathoanatomic confirmation). *J Genet Hum* 21:147–186, 1973.

Petersen I, and Akesson HO. EEG studies of siblings of children showing 14 and 6 per second positive spikes. *Acta Genet* 18:163–169, 1968.

Petrischenko NV. Clinical encephalographic comparisons in families of patients with residual epilepsy. *Zh Nevropat Psikhiatr Korsakov* 68:1599–1604, 1968.

Poch GF, Martin AJ, Zavala HA, and Weinstein IH. Brachymetapoldia associated with epilepsy and migraine. *Pren Med Argent* 57:1744–1745, 1970.

Popova NN, Amadyan MG, and Umanskaya RM. A clinico immunological study of epileptic children, adolescents and their relatives. *Zh Nevropat Psikhiat Korsakov* 75:1194–1197, 1975.

Pryles CV, Livingston S., and Ford FR. Familial paroxysmal choreoathetosis of Mount and Reback. Study of a second family in which this condition is found in association with epilepsy. *Pediatrics* 9:44–47, 1952.

Quattrini A, Marchesi G, and Giuliani G. Clinical and polygraphic study of progressive familial myoclonic epilepsy. Preliminary observations. *Riv Neurol* 45:198–203, 1975.

Radermecker J, and Dumon J. Genetic epilepsies, in Gastaut H, Jasper H, Bancaud J, and Watregney A (eds): *The Physiopathogenesis of the Epilepsies,* Springfield: CC Thomas, 1969, pp 31–35.

Refsum S. Genetics of epilepsies, in Parsonage MJ (ed): *Prevention of Epilepsy and Its Consequences,* The Fifth European Symposium on Epilepsy, held in London, July 17–19, 1972. International Bureau for Epilepsy, London, 1972, pp 11–14.

Richter K. Electroencephalographic findings in relatives of patients with genuine epilepsy. *Arch Psychiatr Nervenkr* 194:443–455, 1956.

Rimoin DL, and Metrakos JD. The genetics of convulsive disorders in the families of hemiplegics. Proceedings of the Second International Congress of Human Genetics, Volume 3, 1963, pp 1655–1658.

Rodin EA. Familial occurrence of the 14 and 6/sec positive spike phenomenon. *Electroencephalogr Clin Neurophysiol* 17:566–570, 1964.

Rodin EA, Doose H, Gerken H, Petersen CE, and Volzke E. The value of EEG Investigations among family members in neurological practice. *Electroencephalogr Clin Neurophysiol* 26:444, 1969.

REFERENCES

Rodin E, and Gonzalez S. Hereditary components in epileptic patients. *JAMA* 198:221–225, 1966.

Rosanoff AJ, Handy LM, and Rosanoff IA: Etiology of epilepsy with special reference to its occurrence in twins. *Arch Neurol Psychiatr* 31:1165–1193, 1934.

Rosenbaum M, and Maltby GC. Cerebral dysrhythmia in relation to eclampsia. *Arch Neurol Psychiatr* 49:204–213, 1943.

Rossini R, Corsino GM, and Lugaresi E. Psychomotor epilepsy during the growth period. *Riv Sper Freniat* 82:7–185, 1958.

Rust J. Genetic effects in the cortical auditory evoked potential: a twin study. *Electroencephalogr Clin Neurophysiol* 39:321–327, 1975.

Sallou C, and Poissonnier M. Familial factors in a population of epileptic adolescents. *Epilepsia* 10:47–54, 1969.

Sasagawa M. A clinico genetical study on the occasions convulsions in young children. *Psychiatr Neurol Jap* 78:217–233, 1976.

Saunders LZ. A check list of hereditary and familial diseases of the central nervous system in domestic animals. *Cornell Vet* 42:592–600, 1952.

Schiøttz-Christensen E. Chorea huntington and epilepsy in monozygotic twins. *Europ Neurol* 2:250–255, 1969.

Schiøttz-Christensen E. Genetic factors in febrile convulsions. An investigation of 64 same sexed twin pairs. *Acta Neurol Scand* 48:538–546, 1972.

Schlesinger K, Boggan W, and Freedman DX. Genetics of audiogenic seizures: I. Relation to brain serotonin and norepinephrine in mice. *Life Sci* 4:2345–2351, 1965.

Seemanova E, Lesny I, Hyanek J et al. X chromosomal recessive microcephaly with epilepsy, spastic tetraplegia and absent abdominal reflexes. New variety of 'Paine syndrome'? *Humangenetik* 20:113–117, 1973.

Segawa M. Congenital muscular dystrophy. *Adv Neurol Sci* 20:68–80, 1976.

Shibasaki H, Kato M, and Kuroiwa Y. Essential myoclonus with paroxysmal electroencephalographic abnormality. Report of a case and electrophysiological study. *Clin Neurol* 13:203–210, 1973.

Shu S. Polyphasic spike or spike and wave complexes occurring in the Rolandic region in children. *J Nagoya Med Assoc* 97:141–146, 1975.

REFERENCES

Skre H. A study of certain traits accompanying some inherited neurological disorders. *Clin Genet* 8:117–135, 1975.

Skre H. Current research in neuroepidemiology. Some main trends. *Acta Neurol Scan* 57 (Suppl 67):11–36, 1978.

Smeraldi E, Scorza-Smeraldi R, Cazzullo CL, Guareschi-Cazzulo A, and Canger R. A genetic approach to the Lennox-Gastaut syndrome by the "Major Histocompatibility Complex" (MHC), in Janz D (ed): *Epileptology,* Proceedings of the Seventh International Symposium on Epilepsy, Berlin (West), June 1975, Thieme, Berlin, 1975, pp 33–37.

Smith B, Robinson GC, and Lennox WG. Acquired epilepsy. (A study of 535 cases.) *Neurology (Minneap)* 4:19–28, 1954.

Sorel L. The descendants of epileptic patients. *Epilepsia* 10:91–96, 1969.

Soulayrol R, Granjon E, Lyagoubi S, Dravet C, and Roger G. Study of familial factors in the population of epileptic children observed at the Saint Paul Centre. *Epilepsia* 10:33–46, 1969.

Stein C. Hereditary factors in epilepsy. A comparative study of 1000 institutionalized epileptics and 1115 non-epileptic controls. *Am J Pediatr* 12:989–1037, 1933.

Stern RS, and Eldridge R. Clinical and genetic study of the progressive myoclonic epilepsies. *Neurology (Minneap)* 23:420, 1973.

Strauss H, Rahm WE Jr, and Barrera SE. Electroencephalographic studies in relatives of epileptics. *Proc Soc Exper Biol Med* 42:207–212, 1939.

Suzuki T. EEG studies on epileptic twins. *Psychiatr Neurol Jap* 62:35–59, 1960.

Szabo L, Durko I, Nagy ME, and Obol F. Biochemical and electroencephalographic investigations in a case of a monozygotic twin pair suffering from phenylketonuria. *Acta Pediatr Acad Sci Hung* 6:227–244, 1965.

Tanaka H, and Aramitsu Y. A survey of epilepsy in infancy and childhood. *Psychiatr Neurol Paediatr Jap* 2:303–310, 1962.

Temkin O. *The Falling Sickness. A History of Epilepsy From The Greeks to the Beginnings of Modern Neurology,* Baltimore: Johns Hopkins Press, 1971.

Thom DA. The relation between the genetic factors and the age of onset in one hundred and fifty seven cases of hereditary epilepsy. *Boston Med Surg J* 173:496–473, 1915.

REFERENCES

Thom DA. A second note on the frequency of epilepsy in the offspring of epileptics. *Boston Med Surg J* 175:599–600, 1916.

Thom DA, and Walker GS. Epilepsy in the offspring of epileptics. *Am J Psychiatr* 1:613–627, 1922.

Tsuboi T. Polygenic inheritance of epilepsy and febrile convulsions: analysis based on a computational model. *Br J Psychiatr* 129:239–242, 1976.

Tsuboi T, and Christian W. On the genetics of the primary generalized epilepsy with sporadic myoclonias of impulsive petit mal type. *Humangenetik* 19:155–182, 1973.

Tsuboi T, and Endo S. Incidence of seizures and EEG abnormalities among offspring of epileptic patients. *Hum Genet* 36:173–189, 1977.

Utin AV. Heterogeneity and several clinico-genetic correlations in epilepsy under inbred conditions. *Genetika* 11:122–131, 1975.

Utin AV. Comparative frequency of phenotypical resemblance of intrafamilial and interfamilial pairs of patients with generalized and focal epilepsy. *Genetika* 11:162–167, 1975.

Van den Berg BJ. Studies on convulsive disorders in young children. IV. Incidence of convulsions among siblings. *Dev Med Child Neurol* 16:457–464, 1974.

Vercelletto P. The hereditary factor in generalized epilepsy. *Int J Ment Health* 1:207–220, 1972.

Vercelletto P, and Courjon J. Hereditary generalized convulsions of early onset. *Concours Med* 89:6273–6290, 1967.

Vercelletto P, and Courjon J. Heredity and generalized epilepsy. *Epilepsia* 10:7–21, 1969.

Vogel F. Genetische aspekte des elektroenzephalogramms. *Dtsch Med Wochenschr* 88:1748–1759, 1963.

Vogel, F. Zur genetischen grundlage fronto-prazentraler β-wellen-gruppen im EEG des menschen. *Humangenetik* 2:227–237, 1966a.

Vogel F. Zur genetischen grundlage occipitaler langsamer β-wellen im EEG des menschen. *Humangenetik* 2:238–245, 1966b.

Vogel F. The EEG of genetically different types of inherited myoclonic epilepsy. *Electroencephalogr Clin Neurophysiol* 26:444, 1969.

Vogel F, and Fujiya Y. The incidence of some inherited EEG variants in normal Japanese and German males. *Humangenetik* 7:38–42, 1969.

Vogel F, Hafner H, and Diebold K. Genetic studies on progressive myoclonus epilepsies. *Humangenetik* 1:437–475, 1965.

REFERENCES

Wada JA. Biochemically induced and genetically determined 'audio-genic' susceptible state, in Barbeau A, and Brunette JR (eds): *Progress in Neuro-Genetics,* Volume I of the Proceedings of the Second International Congress of Neuro-Genetics and Neuro-Ophthalmology of the World Federation of Neurology, Montreal, September 17–22, 1967, Excerpta Medica Foundation, Amsterdam, 1969, pp 689–694.

Wada JA, and Ikeda H. The susceptibility to auditory stimuli of animals treated with methionine sulfoximine. *Exp Neurol* 15:157–165, 1966.

Wakeno M. A family with heredofamilial tremor associated with epileptic disorders. *Psychiatr Neurol Jpn* 77:1–18, 1975.

Walker AE. Post-traumatic epilepsy. *Wld Neurol* 3:185–194, 1962.

Walker AE. A prospectus, in Jasper HH, Ward AA, and Pope A (eds): *Basic Mechanisms of the Epilepsies.* Boston: Little, Brown, 1969, pp 807–814.

Wallace ME. Keeshonds: a genetic study of epilepsy and EEG readings. *J Small Anim Pract* 16:1–10, 1975.

Wasterlain C, and Dhaene R. Familial somatosensory epilepsy. *Acta Neurol Belg* 69:734–742, 1969.

Weiss B, and Badurowa A. Autonomic seizures in Rendu Osler Weber disease. *Neurol Neurochir Pol* 1:409–411, 1967.

Wilson SAK, and Wolfson JM. Organic nervous disease in identical twins. *Arch Neurol Psychiatr* 21:477–490, 1929.

Yoon CH, Petersen JS, and Corrow D. Spontaneous seizures: a new mutation in Syrian golden hamsters. *J Hered* 67:115–116, 1976.

Zeskov P, and Erak P. Etiopathogenic and therapeutic aspects of malignant forms of childhood epilepsy. *Neuropsihiatrija* 20:191–199, 1972.

Znamierowska-Kozik M. The problem of heredity in epilepsy according to electroencephalographic investigations. *Pozn Towarzy Przyjac Nauk, Wyaz Lek,* Prace Kom Med Doswiad, 27:341–370, 1964.

Subject Index

Subject Index